A Brief Introduction to Yoga Philosophy

Based on the Lectures of Srivatsa Ramaswami

Written by

David Hurwitz

The purpose of Yoga is to reduce duḥkha which is caused by avidyā which is annihilated by viveka khyāti which is established by ashtanga yoga which rests on the foundation of yama niyama.

Preface

This little book is for Ramaswami. It is based on his lectures. These are his themes. These are his ideas. And, if I have done my job, you will hear his voice as you read through it.

I first met Srivatsa Ramaswami in 2001 at the SouthWest Yoga conference where he was giving a workshop on Bhakti Yoga. I knew immediately I wanted to study with this man. The knowledge flowed out of him with great depth and generosity. And, he had studied for over three decades with his guru, Sri Krishnamacharya.

And so I did, traveling to Houston on several occasions when he was teaching there for both private and group study. And later bringing him to Los Angeles where he has taught at Loyola Marymount University for the past seven or eight years.

We have since become good friends. It is one of the joys of my life.

At Loyola he has taught a course on the Yoga Sutras of Patañjali several times now. This book is based principally on two of those courses: the one taught in 2006 and the other in 2008. I have been able to supplement these courses with material I learned from many private sessions I have had with Ramaswami.

Ramaswami has been kind enough to read through the entire manuscript and make corrections for accuracy. Of course, whatever errors remain are my responsibility alone.

The goal of Yoga is to come to know the true nature of the Self. This Self, as Radhakrishnan puts it, is deep below the plane of our empirical life of imagination, will and feeling. It is the ultimate being of man, his true center, which remains unmoved and unchanged, even when on the surface we have the fleeting play of thoughts and emotions, hopes and desires.

And, "where" do we find this Self? According to the seers who gave us the Upanishads, we find the Self abiding in the secret place of the heart, in the lotus of the heart, in The Sky in the Heart.

Contents

Preface..3

Introduction..6

1 The Goal..12

2 Sāṁkhya: Prakriti and the Gunas...........................24

3 The First Step: Kriya Yoga.....................................41

4 The Kleśas..49

5 Duḥkha (Pain)..61

6 Aṣṭāṅga Yoga – The Means.....................................67

7 Yama Niyama...76

8 Āsana...93

9 Prānāyāma...101

10 Pratyāhāra...119

11 Antaraṅga Sādhana (meditation)..........................125

12 Transformation (Pariṇāma)..................................141

Biblography...150

Introduction

This is a small book about Yoga Philosophy. Which means this is a small book about the Yoga Sutras of Patañjali.

Yoga Sutra

Of all the textural studies of Yoga the most important is the Yoga Sutra of Patañjali. Perhaps 2000 years old, the text was written in the sutra form. This is a highly compressed form that facilitated memorization. There were no printed books back then, only oral transmission. Each sutra would then be expanded on by the teacher to a full discussion of its topic. The result was a comprehensive presentation of Yoga. But the text itself was dense and cryptic. The sutras themselves are without verbs. For these reasons the YS is a difficult text to read without accompanying commentary or teacher. Yet, as regards Yoga it is considered authoritative.

Overview of YS

The YS is written in four chapters:

Chapter I. Different kinds of Samādhi. Chapter I is for the advanced yogi. (As Vyasa puts it in his commentary at the start of Chapter II, The Yoga attained by a Yogin with a mind capable of Samadhi has been stated.)

Chapter II. Means to reach Samādhi for those who are not already capable of that state.

Chapter III. What can be accomplished with the mind once you are able to achieve Samādhi.

Chapter IV. Nature of freedom.

Commentaries on YS

There have been many commentaries written on the YS. The two we refer to occasionally are by Vyasa and Hariharānanda. The commentary of Vyasa was probably written a few centuries after Patañjali and is the oldest extant commentary we have. It is regarded by most as authoritative. The one by Hariharānanda is almost contemporary, written in the first half of the 20th century.

While we go into the meaning of many Sanskrit words this is not a word by word translation. It may be helpful to have a word by word or at least a sutra by sutra translation available as you read through this text. Two translations we recommend are the one by Saṁkhya master Hariharānada Āranya which includes the commentary of Vyasa and the word by word translation of Pam Hoxsey following the lectures of Ramaswami.

The Word Yoga

The common meaning of Yoga is union. In Haṭha Yoga it is the union of prāna and apāna; in the Yoga Yajnavalkya it is uniting with God, the union of the jīvātmān with paramātman. However in Patañjali the word Yoga does not mean union. In Patañjali Yoga means Samadhi or concentration. More precisely, Patañjali defines Yoga as nirodha or nirodha Samadhi i.e., the balance of the three gunas or peace of mind. This is the definition he gives in his famous second sutra.

Reality

Unlike some Indian philosophies, e.g. Advaita Vedanta, in which the world is considered to be an illusion, in Yoga the world is real. In fact in Yoga there are three tattvas or principles or reals. They are Purusha or pure consciousness, Prakriti or nature or the world (which includes the mind and the senses) and Īśvara or the Lord or God (though in Yoga he is not a creator God).

Saṁkhya

From Saṁkhya, the underlying philosophy accepted by Patañjali, come the concepts of Puruṣa, Prakṛti and the three Gunas. Puruṣa means the indwelling principle. It is the observer in us. It is pure consciousness and non-changing. Prakṛti is that which evolves. It has three fundamental constituent characteristics known as the gunas. They are sattva which is lightness at the physical level and clarity at the mental level; rajas which is restless physical activity and mental instability; and tamas which is heaviness at the physical level and inertia at the mental level.

The main text of the Saṁkhya philosophy is the Saṁkhya Kārikā of Īśvara Kṛṣṇa.

Purpose

The goal of this little book is to be a guide along the path of Yoga for the average practitioner. We take the definition of Yoga to be Chitta Vritti Nirodha as stated by Patañjali in his famous second sutra.

The purpose of this book is not to convert the YS into a self-help manual or a guide for daily living, though many have done just that. There are, of course, many benefits for life and living which accrue to the practitioner who travels along the path of Yoga. Not least of which are peace and clarity (sattva) of mind and health and lightness of body. Indeed Patañjali's understanding of mind is so deep that many of his, or rather Yoga's, insights can be extremely helpful in our daily struggle to be human. But we do not view this as the raison d'etre for which Patañjali. wrote his sutras.

In fact there is an inherent tension between the path of Yoga and everyday living. For most of daily life the mind travels out through the senses to encounter the world (vyuthita) whereas in Yoga practice we try to create an inward experience, to withdraw the mind from the senses and focus on ever subtler principles. The mind can go in two directions, outward or inward.

One of the fundamental concepts of Yoga is samskāra or mental habit. All of Yoga is concerned with transformation of the mind. This means changing our samskāras. One of the transformations we want to make is from outgoing samskāras to inward samskāras. Daily life creates, supports, and strengthens our outgoing samskāras whereas the Yoga we practice seeks to replace these with samskāras which focus the mind inward. These two are in conflict.

But who among us is going to run off and live in some cave or head into the woods and practice Yoga 24/7? Only one in a million, or perhaps one in a billion, is going to become a true Yogi.

Still our purpose here is to describe the true path of the Yogi.

Technical Note

This technical note is meant for those already familiar with the YS. Of course, experts are not supposed to read this book at all. But, as a statement like that may prove a temptation, let me explain.

How this book is brief? This book is brief by way of being practical. By focusing on what is of immediate import to the average practitioner we have been able to make certain strategic omissions from the YS.

Thus, we have begun with Chapter I sutras 1-4 which give the goal of the text. Then we omitted the rest of Chapter I which is intended for the advanced Yogi. That is, Chapter I is meant for the Yogi who already has a stable mind. For the rest of us, those of us who have distracted minds – which means most of us -- we move directly into Chapter II. We have included a brief summary of Saṁkhya, namely Prakriti and the Guna theory so that we could omit Patañjali's restatement of this material in Chapter II. Then, from Chapter II we have included the Kriya Yoga section, but omitted the theory of karma (YS II.12, 13, 14, 16). Next is the main bulk of our text, the presentation of Astanga Yoga from Chapter II and the beginning of Chapter III is included, but the siddhis of YamaNiyama are omitted. We conclude with the sutras on transformation from Chapter III. We then omit the rest of Chapter III on the siddhis and all of Chapter IV.

Words and Meaning

Words are of limited use when we're talking about the infinite or the eternal or what lies beyond the senses. Words can serve merely as indicators or pointers. But we have to use them. What else do we have? In the end there is only the practice, only the Yoga.

"Words and mind go to him, but reach him not and return."

--- Taittirya Upanishad

Who is This Book For?

This book is for you – if you are a Yoga student or practitioner who has begun a Yoga practice and wishes now to go a bit deeper in your understanding.

It is for you if you have encountered a bit of Yoga Philosophy and want a bit more.

It is for you if you have heard the YS referred to and want to see if you have a taste for it.

It is for you if you want some guidance as to what the goals and methods of Yoga really are.

1

The Goal

Traditional Yoga

Often in classical Indian texts the goal of the text is stated first. So it is with the YS. The essence, goal, and meaning of the entire subject of Yoga are stated in the first four sutras of Chapter One. For those advanced enough to understand and practice it, nothing else is needed.

The first sutra (I.1) of the YS is, "Now I am going to talk about Yoga." Here Patañjali announces the subject of his text: Yoga. But not just Yoga. In this sutra he uses the Sanskrit word "anuṡāsanam". "anu" means "follows"; and "ṡāsanam" means "that which is well established, authoritative." Thus the meaning of the word "anuṡāsanam" in the sutra is: that which follows the well established or authoritative texts or that which is consistent with tradition, meaning the Vedas.

So, the meaning of the sutra becomes: Now a text on Yoga which follows authoritative tradition. Patañjali does not claim to have written an original text. Rather he claims to have collected, collated, and rewritten well established traditional texts that follow the authority of the Vedas.

The YS of Patañjali is <u>the</u> text of traditional Yoga. Any other text or teaching or practice can and should be measured against the yardstick of Patañjali. If it is in agreement with Patañjali then it is in accord with traditional Yoga. If it conflicts or violates Patañjali then it is not traditional Yoga.

At the time of Patañjali other practices were being promulgated as Yoga. Many were not following tradition. (Certain tantric practices are examples.) And, as a result tradition was being corrupted. One motivation Patañjali may have had for writing the YS was to re-establish just what was traditional Yoga. For only by following the path of traditional Yoga you will achieve the goal that is promised. It is not possible otherwise.

The Five States of Mind

According to Vyasa's commentary on I.1 the mind can be in any one of five states:

1. kṣipta: completely shattered, restless. Such minds are completely broken. They cannot be repaired.

2. mūḍha: addicted to going out through the senses; completely infatuated. It can derive happiness only through the senses. I've got to see good things, hear good things, smell good things, touch good things. If I don't have the objects to excite me and give me pleasure I am unhappy.

3. vikṣhipta: sometimes focused, sometimes distracted. This is the state most of us are in most of the time. For most of us this is the normal state. Why don't I try Yoga, why don't I try this, why don't I try that. Despite all the good things that I have there is an undercurrent of unhappiness.

4. Ekāgra: the mind is capable of remaining focused. This is the one pointed state in which the same object is kept in the mind moment after moment. Some people have this capability naturally.

5. Nirodha: arrested state in which the activities of the mind are stopped completely. There is total satisfaction. This is a state of the mind we are not aware of. We cannot even imagine this.

Only the last two, ekāgra and nirodha, are considered states of Yoga.

We are not aware of the fifth state and we are not aware of the first state. Generally, our minds wander around among states two, three and four.

Those in the first two states are not capable of taking up the practice of Yoga. In the kṣipta state they cannot follow an instruction and do not have the patience or intelligence necessary for contemplation. Those in the mūḍha state are addicted to sensory pleasures. They are totally infatuated and so have no desire to do Yoga or think on subtle principles. But, those in the vikṣhipta state can focus their minds some of the time. They can intellectually understand subtle principles when they are described in Yoga texts, but are constantly distracted. These are the people who can practice Yoga. For them, Yoga practice can remove the distractions of the mind. Over time, Yoga can bring their minds to the Ekāgra or even the Nirodha state. Every mind is capable of that.

Mechanics of perception

In sutra I.2 Patañjali defines Yoga using three technical words: Chitta, Vritti, and Nirodha. Chitta is the mind or brain. This comes from Cit which means consciousness and Chitta meaning that which appears to have consciousness, that which masquerades as consciousness. Vritti is a word which is notoriously hard to translate. It normally means activity and here refers to our mental activities or projections. Nirodha is to stop completely. This comes from ni, permanently, and rodha, to stop. Here it means stoppage of all the mental activities. A state in which the mind has come to rest.

When we "see" an object outside us what happens? Light rays from the object enter our eyes, impact our retina, and are converted into nerve impulses which are then "interpreted" by the brain as the outside object.

In effect, the mind projects an image of the object onto our mental space. This mental projection is called a "vritti". The citta akasha, or mental space, is created by the mind -- just as it does when we dream. The mind projects the object onto our citta akahsa as though the object were outside the mind. This vritti is not merely a visual projection, but a composite including sound, temperature, etc. And, we get a feeling that these are coming from outside.

Not only that, the mind also projects "me", as though I'm sitting in front of the object and observing it. Vritti refers to the whole composite projection. What I normally consider to be "me" -- the mind-body complex, the personality, the ego, the twenty year old "me" or the sixty year old "me", the "me" that is sometimes happy and sometimes sad -- is just part of the experienced world. That is, "me" is included in the object.

Mental Activities – Chitta Vrittis

These mental projections are the chitta vrittis. They are not just what we perceive or take in through the senses. One moment the mind may project something we see, the next moment I may close my eyes and project something from the past, the next it may be something I imagine, etc.

The mind may also project a feeling or emotion based on a perception or a memory or a dream or something I imagine. I may be frightened or hopeful, happy or unhappy. These are all vrittis as well.

In fact anything and everything that I am experiencing at a particular moment is a chitta vritti.

But this is by no means the whole story on vrittis. For more see pps. 8-9 of YBS, pps. 42-6 of YTSL, and the commentary of Vyasa and Hariharananda on sutras I.5-11 in HA.)

The Self

But if what I normally consider to be "me" is just another object in the mental plane then who is observing this "me" looking at the object? I know when I am happy; I know when I am unhappy. If these are known there must be something else doing the knowing. There must be some principle observing. Yoga insists on such a principle.

When I was a young man this principle was observing what I call "me". When I am an old man this principle is observing what I call "me". When I am older the mind has changed. What was pleasurable then may not be pleasurable now. What I thought then I may not think now. My body has certainly undergone changes. In other words, what I call "me" has undergone changes. Yet we feel the principle that observes the young "me" and the older "me" has stayed the same. This principle has not undergone any change. It has remained a constant. This Yoga calls "I".

"I" is called the Drasta or the Seer or the Self or pure consciousness or awareness or Purusha or the indwelling principle. The Seer is unwavering, constant. It does not undergo any change. It is beyond time. It is eternal. It is immortal. In each and every one of us the true Self is immortal.

Now I realize that I am the observer of my mental projections. The Self observes all the chitta vrittis projected by the mind. Purusha experiences everything that goes on in the mind. I am not just the physical person sitting and writing. I am the one who is aware of the changing projections of my mind. I am the one who has always been aware of the changing projections of my mind.

The subject is the Self which is pure awareness; the object is my chitta vrittis. And, the chitta vrittis consist of the empirical self (what I normally call "me"), the senses, and the objects of experience.

The Purusha or the Self does not see the outside world. It sees only what is projected by the mind.

Purusha need not be seen to be known. In fact it is subtle, beyond the senses.

Definition of Yoga

In sutra I.2 Patañjali defines Yoga as "chitta vritti nirodhaḥ." Yoga is the complete stoppage of the mental activities or projections. Here vritti is plural. It represents all the mental activities. We may perceive something with the senses, look at one thing and imagine another, think of the past, sleep, etc. There are many vrittis. Yoga is the stoppage of all of them.

Stop here does not mean to forcibly stop. It is not due to an external force. Rather you have to work the mind in such a way that it will come to a standstill by itself. You create the conditions that allow the mind to naturally come to a stop of its own accord. If a truck is racing downhill the only way to stop it is to get into the truck and apply the brake. Likewise you must get into your own mind and stop it. You make use of your own mind to stop the mind. The way of doing this, as stated in the YS, is by coming to know the true nature of the Self.

Sometimes our minds do come to a stop. For example, we may see a beautiful sunset. One that takes our breath away. For a few moments, we may have no thoughts or feelings. We lose ourselves in the beauty of the sunset. Then the moment passes and our minds start up again. This is not Yoga. For we are not in control. Indeed, we may return in a few days to another beautiful sunset only to find the experience does not recur.

Normally, the mind recognizes all our various desires and we go about trying to satisfy them. As we all learn sooner or later this does not work. Satisfying desires simply leads to more desires. Our own mind becomes the runaway truck. On the other hand, by knowing the true nature of the Self the mind realizes that what it has been doing is not really necessary. For the Self is already in a state of total satisfaction. And then, when this realization comes, the mind automatically arrives at Nirodha, the final stage.

According to Yoga every mind has the capability to transform from distraction to ekagra to Nirodha – provided we have the interest and motivation and take the steps necessary i.e. practice Yoga.

One more thing. Since the brain also is responsible for maintaining life a question arises. If all the activities of the mind are stopped does that mean life also will come to an end? The answer is no. The reason is given in the Sāṁkhya text. There they say there are two kinds of vrittis. Here we are only concerned with the thought activities. But there are also other vrittis, namely those maintaining our physiological activities. Those vrittis which maintain our physiological activities are known as samanya vrittis or common vrittis. The brain has two functions, chitta vrittis and samanya vrittis. When Patañjali talks about the chitta vrittis he is talking only about the mental activities, not the physiological activities.

So Yoga is the stopping of the chitta vritti or a state in which the mind comes to a complete rest.

Benefits of Yoga

If the mind stops what is the benefit? Complete peace. There is a continual flow of peace (called praśāntavāhitā in Sanskrit) in the mind. "flow" here means that moment after moment there is peace. Moment after moment the mind is in the same state.

Here "peace" means the three gunas of the mind have returned to a state of equilibrium. The mind does not present any experience to the Purusha. There is no excitement or happiness or bliss or any kind of feeling. The mind is perfectly clear. It is like a crystal without a flaw. The mind is in a state of absolute peace. This is a state we have no awareness of. This is a state we cannot even imagine.

When the chitta vrittis are gone what remains? Drasta, the observer. Once the mind settles down, the Self or Puruṣa remains in its own form. The purusha is free of all chitta vrittis. This is real freedom.

Quieting the Mind

Why won't the mind settle down and be quiet? Because of our samskaras, our habits. Maybe we've read about the goal of Yoga in the YS or some other book, but just because we know the goal of Yoga intellectually does not mean the mind will settle down (though this is the right first step). Just because we read the YS and learn that Yoga is chitta vritti nirodha does not mean that we can close our eyes and be there. Why? Because of our samskaras. We have been following the same mental habits, samskaras, day after day, year after year, all our life until now. They don't change overnight. They tend to continue as they always have. If we want to change our samskaras we have to put in the effort. Yoga is all about changing our samskaras. Yoga is all about transforming our mind.

Why does the mind settle down? Because it knows the true nature of the Self. We are always trying to please the pseudo-self, the mind-body complex that we mistakenly think is the Self. We think the pseudo-self is who we are. We want to feel happy; not feel pain. We constantly work toward this goal by trying to please the pseudo-self. The pseudo-self is real. It exists. But it is not the Self. It is not who we really are. And once the mind realizes this pseudo-self is not the Self, the mind settles down.

In Sāṁkhya the example of the dancer and the King is given. The dancer dances to please the King. She tries every movement and technique she knows. Until one day she realizes the King doesn't care. He's just sitting there watching. Then, of course, she stops dancing.

So it is with the mind and the true Self. The true Self is already satisfied. It does not require any of the things we are doing to feel satisfied.

The parallel is in dream. The dream space is projected. The dream objects are projected. The dream self is projected. And, the mind identifies with that self, the dream self. Then there is the dream experience.

Just as when we get up in the morning we realize the dream self is a false self, so also when we realize the pseudo-self is not the real Self, but only a mental projection, then we wake up. Not that the world is unreal. Patañjali doesn't say that. For Yoga takes the world to be real. Rather just as in the dream where we identify with the dream self and forget about the dreamer, Patañjali says that we have forgotten about our true Self. The dream self and the pseudo-self are both chitta vrittis. They are both false, not the true Self.

So how do we proceed on this quest to know the true nature of the Self? There are three steps.

1. The first stage is understanding at the intellectual level. You listen to what Patañjali has to say. You hear his ideas. You hear a different way of looking at things. There is a germ of an idea which starts to grow in your own mind. This is called paroksha. You hear it from another person. You get paroksha jnanam through an authority like Patañjali. But, of course, this is someone else's experience.

2. The second stage is to become convinced. You read some more books. You talk it over with your friends. You question and try and find out what is wrong with the ideas. You keep on thinking about it over and over again. Slowly it starts building in your mind. Ultimately you are convinced. This stage is known as anumana. Finally, when all the doubts have been answered, you come to your own conclusion, your own conviction. Still, it is not sufficient.

3. You do the appropriate practice. Only then does the necessary transformation take place in your mind. You develop a one pointed mind. You get into the state of Samadhi. You're able to directly perceive it. That is, direct yogic perception which differs from ordinary perception. Only then does chitta vritti nirodha happen. This is possible only through Yoga. Yogic procedures are necessary because these ideas are subtle. They can't be seen. They can't be heard. They can't be perceived by the senses.

When the mind is quiet

Then Tadā draṣṭuḥ svarūpe avasthānam. The Self remains in its own form.

When that happens then the mind is able to realize that the true Self is the observer which does not undergo any change. Then the mind no longer projects "me" as the Self. The emphasis shifts. The objects are the projections of my mind; the subject is the Purusha or the Self. In the ekagrata state there is only one object: the projection of my mind. And, there is an observer called Purusha or the Self. The subject is the Observer; the object is my chitta vritti.

Nirodha means no chitta vrittis. Nirodha means completely surrounding something. Citta vṛitti nirodhaḥ means the mind is not allowed to escape. In the state of nirodha the Purusha will not experience or observe anything. No pleasure; no pain. There is only Purusha. The mind is in a state of absolute peace.

What happens when the mind is not quiet?

On all other occasions, because the mind does not know the true nature of the Self, it will create a pseudo-self. The pseudo-self we call "me". It identifies with this mind-body complex, with this personality, this particular person. And, the mind keeps on working to make this particular person happy.

In sutra I.3 Patañjali uses the word svarūpe which means one's own form; in sutra I.4 he uses the word sārūpyaṁ which means one which looks like this. The mind is able to create another self (the way dream creates a dream self). It creates something which is similar to the Self, a poor copy of the Self. It is not the original. It is not the real thing. And, then the mind identifies this created self, this "me", as the Self. Sārūpyaṁ means the mind creates another self, a false self, with which it is able to identify. The mind cannot function without a self. That is why it creates one.

The one who experiences everything should be called I. And this, Patañjali says, is the consciousness. It is absolutely distinct from anything I experience. I experience "me". I experience that I exist. But nothing that is experienced can be the true Self. Anything that is experienced is not the Self

2

Sāṁkhya: Prakṛti and the Gunas

Prakriti

The body, the mind, and the senses are all part of Prakriti. Only the Purusha is not part of Prakriti. According to Sāṁkhya there are 24 principles (tattvas) which do not belong to the Self. These 24 principles make up Prakrti. They are: mulaprakriti, mahat tattva/buddhi, ahamkara, manas, 5 jnana indriyas, 5 karma indriyas, the 5 tanmatras, and the 5 gross elements.

The mulaprakriti with the three gunas is in a state of equilibrium. This is the starting point. This is Nature. It evolves into this universe. Like the big bang singularity in Physics.

Evolution (SK 22 – 29)

Evolution according to Sāṁkhya starts with Satva dominating. Out of mulaprakriti arises the first principle: Mahat tattva, the great principle. This is the first stage of evolution. It is normally associated with the Universal Intelligence. The Sāṁkhyas believe the mahat tattva, the universal intelligence, is necessary for creating the universe. Some coordinating principle is necessary.

Note that intelligence is not part of consciousness. This is because intelligence can be known. Intelligence can be experienced. Therefore it is not the Self or consciousness. The same is true for manas or mind.

Next to evolve is the ahaṃkāra tattva. The ego. This is due to rajasic evolution. This universal ego is also necessary for creation of the universe. There needs to be a motivation. Mere intelligence is not sufficient. Knowing how to create the universe is not enough. A motivation is needed. And, that is produced by ahamkara.

The ahamkara also produces individuals.

Out of this ahamkara there are two streams of evolution: microcosmic (the individual) and macrocosmic (the universe). The microcosmic arises out of satvic evolution; the macrocosmic comes out of tamasic evolution.

Then why do we call ahaṃkāra rajasic evolution? Because rajas energizes both Sattva and Tamas which by themselves are inert and incapable of performing any function. Thus, rajas is instrumental in the evolution of both the microcosmic and the macrocosmic. It excites Sattva and Tamas to perform their own activities.

Microcosmic Evolution: the Indriyas

The microcosmic level (these are inside us):

The five jnana Indriyas (the senses): eyes, ears, nose, tongue, skin.

The five karma Indriyas (by which we act): speech, arms, legs, excretory organ, generative organ.

Manas, or mind, the coordinating indriya. When you hear something or see something all of the input goes into your mind. The mind is the one that controls. It is the coordinating agency called manas.

These are the eleven indriyas.

Macrocosmic Evolution: Tanmatras and the bhutas

At the macrocosmic level:

The five tanmatras. sound, touch, form, taste, smell.

From the five tanmatras evolve the five bhutas (elements):

From sabda (sound) evolves space
From sparsa (touch) evolves air
From rupa (form) evolves fire
From rasa (taste) evolves water
From ganda (smell) evolves earth

Objects are made up of these five elements.

These 24 principles are the principles with which the entire universe is created

All the 24 tattvas are not the Self. Because everything is experienced. I experience every one of these as a chitti vritti.

How the Indriyas Work

If these elements are to be grasped by the indriyas, (you can't directly grasp space, etc.), they will have to be grasped through the tanmatras. The tanmatras impinge on the respective indriyas. The sound (sabda) tanmatra impinges on your ears. The rupa (form) tanmatra impinges on your eyes. This is akin to light particles coming from the object.

How do I see? Only by the tanmatras coming. When I see a particular object that object remains there. I get only light out of that. Likewise if someone makes a noise only the sound comes to us.

The five bhutas are there. But the indriyas do not collect the bhutas, only the tanmatras.

The macrocosmic world and the microcosmic are related when the indriyas are able to get the tanmatras. That is how we perceive the outside world.

The senses receive all the information. The manas coordinates the senses. Then the ego comes in. When I get a lot of information immediately there is a feeling: I like this; I don't like this. And then, the whole thing is presented to the buddhi.

Patañjali and Sāṁkhya

Patañjali in his Yoga accepts the Sāṁkhya Philosoply, but does not specify the 24 principles. He rather divides them into four groups: viśeṣa, aviśeṣa, lingamātra, and alinga. Instead of saying the five gross principles, he puts it into one, the Vitarkas.

Gunas (SK 12,13)

Origin of the Gunas

What is the original source of the three gunas? The three gunas are already mentioned in the Vedas.

Meaning of Guna

Guna has two meanings which are important for Yoga. One meaning is strand; the other is a characteristic. Guna means a strand or a characteristic. These two meanings are used by the ancient philosophers of Sāṁkhya and Yoga.

Universe Made from Gunas

Supposing you've got three strands or threads. One is white, one is black, and one is red. You twist them into a twine. And, then you give it to a weaver. He can make an enormous number of patterns, different fabrics, different clothing with the twine. But basically they are all made of these threads – a black strand, a white strand, and a red strand.

Sāṁkhya takes this example and says the entire universe is nothing but different patterns made up of these three gunas. White refers to Satva, red to rajas, and black to Tamas.

White is purity, satva. Red is rajas. The moment you see red you get excited. Red is associated with activity. And, black is associated with Tamas, inactivity, inertia, gloom, etc.

These three put together form the entire universe. Everything can be broken down into the satvic component, the rajasic component, the tamasic component.

It is very difficult to separate rajas, tamas, and satva. The only way we know them is we are able to see their effects.

Gunas in the Individual

How do the gunas manifest in the individual? All three gunas are in us, but normally one guna dominates us. The other two gunas are subservient to the main guna.

Yoga is primarily about reducing rajas and tamas and making satva more and more dominant. In the ultimate state all the gunas are in a state of equilibrium.

More than their effect on the outside world, in Yoga we are concerned with the effect of these three qualities on us. Our mind and body change depending on which quality predominates in us. What quality predominates depends on our samskaras.

If I had rajasic tendencies when I was young and continue to operate in the same mold then rajas will be the dominant guna all my life. Because rajas feeds rajas I get into that groove: excessive energy, fickle mind, anger, etc. As I do rajasic activities the rajasic samskaras get strengthened. The angry young man becomes the angry old man. Likewise if I am a satvic person I will continue to be satvic; if tamasic I will continue to be tamasic.

Normally, if you don't do anything about it these gunas don't change. But Patañjali and the Yoga say that it is possible to change which guna predominates. A tamasic person can become a rajasic person by the appropriate practices. A rajasic person can become a satvic person. I can change the samskaras. I can change the mental makeup itself. For that the Yogic methods are suggested. These transformations are known as parinamas in Sanskrit. A topic we will come back to later.

In the Bhagavad Gita Lord Krishna tells Arjuna: if you are a tamasic person become a rajasic person. A tamasic person is dull, weak, not doing any activity. Become a rajasic person – that means start doing something. Begin an activity to get out of this tamasic mold. Then, if you are a rajasic person become a satvic person. That is the next thing Lord Krishna says. Become more and more contemplative. Then, if you are a satvic person go beyond the three gunas. This is what is known as chitta vritti nirodhah. Where all the three gunas are in a state of equilibrium.

Rajas and tamas easily overshadow satva. Only a small percentage of people are satvic, most have a predominance of rajas or tamas.

Sattva in the Individual

How can you know that something is satvic? Satva is lightness in the physical body; and clarity at the mental level. When the satva guna is dominant in us then we find its effects. If you are satvic then at the physical level you feel lightness. If you get up in the morning and you feel light then that morning you are satvic. It could be because you ate satvic food or got a good night's rest, etc. There are some people who feel light in the morning most of the time. Such people are satvic. From the time they wake up til the time they get out of bed is very short. They get out of bed as soon as they wake up. Satva at the mental level means clarity. Satvic people have a very clear mind. You tell them something and immediately they are able to understand. They are able to understand a lot of things more quickly than most of us. So, if a person is satvic, at the physical level he is light and mentally he is very clear. In Sāṁkhya this is the most desirable quality.

If you feel light physically and are very clear in your mind and if this state continues moment after moment you are in a satvic mold. If I want my mind to have more and more clarity I should make my mind more and more satvic.

People who are satvic have an undercurrent of peace in them. They are dharmic. They do whatever has to be done. Satva is associated with peace. Unfortunately most of us are in a rajasic mold because of our desire for acquisitions.

A satvic person can go in any one of four directions.

A satvic person has an orderly mind. He knows right from wrong. He can follow a path of dharma. That is, he is clear about what should be done and what should not be done. That is called dharma.

A satvic person is able to understand the spiritual truths.

He can become more and more detached, a recluse.

Or he is able to attain supernatural powers. It comes to satvic people naturally.

Rajas in the Individual

On the other hand, if you are in a rajasic mold then there is a physical restlessness. If rajas is the predominant guna, you engage in a lot of excessive physical activity. You can't sit still. You have to constantly be physically active.

They give the example of a bull. When a bull sees another bull it immediately charges, starting a bullfight. That is the natural tendency of a bull. The bull is a very rajasic animal. People who are very rajasic tend to get into confrontations with other people.

At the mental level, the mind is fickle, restless. It is not able to focus or concentrate on anything. It will be with an object for a moment, next moment it will move to something else, third moment another object which may not be related to the first object. The mind jumps from one object to another. A chain of thoughts. Or rather a train of thoughts, one car after another. Each is different.

People who are rajasic are usually unhappy. There is a lot of pain. Because you keep on trying to acquire things. This requires a lot of effort for which you get a fleeting moment of pleasure.

Tamas in the Individual

In the tamasic mold, if tamas is predominant in you, there is heaviness of the body, heaviness at the physical level. A tamasic person takes a long time to get out of the bed. They are phlegmatic. You may feel sleepy. Perhaps because you ate heavy food. When you are tamasic you are dull and lazy. You tend to sleep.

At the mental level, there is a covering, like a veil. Nothing gets into the mind. There is complete darkness, a lack of clarity.

They say people who are tamasic are deluded. They don't take care of anything. They don't take care of themselves; they don't take care of their families. Depression is tamasic. Depression is daurmanasya, a weak mind, a mind which will not fight. Hence tamasic.

The tamasic person is the opposite of the satvic person. You become adharmic, doing that which is not proper. Tamasic people become so entangled with the pleasures and pains of the body that sensual pleasure is their only goal. They get pleasure only through the senses. "I want this, I want that." There is no question of dispassion. They become slaves. Slaves to other people; slaves to different ideas; slaves to the senses.

Physical Location of the Gunas in the Individual

If we look at our own body, the neck and above is called satvic. From neck to navel is the rajasic portion. Below that is the tamasic portion.

Yoga and the Gunas

The Bhagavad Gita, Sāṁkhya, and some Upanishads all talk about reducing rajas and tamas so satva will be the dominant guna, but it is only in Yoga that practical methods are given to reduce the tamo and rajo gunas. There if you are a rajasic person the practice of asana is suggested. If one practices asana over a period of time the rajas comes down.

But this is not sufficient because the mental space which has been vacated by rajas can be taken over by tamas. But, as is said in the YS, by the practice of pranayama the veil or covering of tamas is reduced.

That is why in the olden days you always practiced asana and pranayama together.

By the practice of asana rajas comes down; by the practice of pranayama tamas comes down. Satva becomes dominant. Then you are in a better position to use your satvic mind for meditation. Only a satvic mind can meditate. A tamasic mind cannot meditate. It will go to sleep. A rajasic mind cannot meditate because it will be fluctuating. It will not be able to focus attention on an object.

If you are a rajasic or tamasic person and you try to meditate without asana and pranayama you will not succeed. If you are already a satvic person perhaps you don't need asana and pranayama.

The Five States of the Mind and the Three Gunas

From the point of view of the Yogi, we can explain the states of Yoga with the three gunas.

The three gunas have different characteristics and are opposed to each other. One is clarity, one is lack of clarity, one is energy. Satva is associated with order (dharma), tamas with chaos. Sometimes the mind is very orderly. In that case it is satvic. Sometimes the mind is absolutely chaotic. That means it is in a tamasic mold.

Because of the predominance of one guna or the other things keep on changing. When satva dominates everything is clear. I attend a class and I'm able to understand everything. Another day I don't understand anything. The reason is that on that day I'm in a tamasic mold. Tamas is predominant at that particular time.

All three gunas work in unison even though they are opposed to each other.

Let's look at the three gunas with respect to our own mind. How do we explain the five states of the mind with the three gunas? The five states are kshipta, mudha, vikshipta, ekagrata, and the ultimate state, nirodha.

When the mind of an individual is predominantly rajasic then it is in a state of kshipta. Absolutely out of control. E.g., when I'm angry, agitated. For some people this is their first reaction whenever there is a problem. They get angry.

The second state is mudha, completely infatuated. Spending all your time trying to gratify the senses. I keep on eating; I keep on listening to music; I keep on watching tv. The way I get pleasure is through the senses. This is a tamasic mold.

Most of us are not in these two states. We sometimes get angry. We sometimes get confused. We sometimes like to enjoy with our senses. Sometimes we are able to concentrate. This is the third state, called Vikshipta, in which the three gunas alternate. Sometimes I'm satvic; sometimes rajasic; sometimes tamasic. For these people the three gunas keep on alternating.

The fourth state is called ekagrata. A mind which is satvic is able to focus very easily. A satvic mind is able to concentrate on one thing even though there are other disturbances. Whereas in the Vikshipta state we are easily distracted. When you are able to focus your understanding of the object you are contemplating on becomes better. That leads to samprajnata Samadhi where the mind is totally focused on the object and everything that is to be known about the object is completely known to you. Like some of the scientists who are able to concentrate completely. Or people who make great music. They are totally with the object. Some get it naturally, due to previous samskaras. Some get it by birth.

The fifth state is nirodha. Here the gunas are in a state of equilibrium. No one of them is predominant. Satva also comes down because there is nothing further for satva to do. The ultimate goal has been reached. So, it settles down.

In the first state, second state, and the fourth state one of the three gunas is predominant. In the third state they are equally powerful. In the ultimate (5th) state all of them are in equilibrium. In this way we can relate the gunas with the five mental states.

To summarize:

The three Gunas and the five levels (bhumi) of the mind (chitta) according to Yogic understanding:

1. People whose minds are fragmented/demonic (kshipa) are predominantly Rajasic.
2. People whose minds are infatuated with sense objects (mudha) are predominantly Tamasic.
3. People whose minds are distracted now, focused then (vikshipta) have their mind flip-flop among Satwic, Rajasic and Tamasic states.
4. People who have well focused minds (ekagra) are basically Satwic.
5. Yogis in a state of absolute Freedom or Kaivalya/ have their minds in total peace (Nirodha) may be said to be in a state in which all three Gunas are in perfect equilibrium (Samya avastha).

The Goal of Yoga and the Gunas

What Yoga does is change the pattern of vikshipta, the state most of us are normally in in which the balance of the gunas keeps on changing, to a state in which the mind becomes predominantly satvic.

That is what we want to achieve. That is what the first goal of Yoga is. Because with a satvic mind I can achieve all the things that are mentioned in Yoga. The achievement of the various Yogic siddhis, including the knowledge of the true nature of the self, becomes possible when my mind becomes satvic.

Most of the spiritual matters mentioned in the Yoga texts, like the nature of the Self, don't appear to be clear when my mind is disturbed. We need a lot of time without the mind wandering. Only a mind which does not wander will be able to focus. That is possible only when my mind is satvic.

The Practice of Yoga and the Gunas

Yoga gives us a means for achieving this. How? The first five angas, yama, niyama, asana, pranayama, pratyahara are there to reduce the rajas and tamas in us so that satva becomes the predominant quality. The texts say that asana reduces the rajo guna. Then pranayama reduces the tamo guna. This is why we try and do both asana and pranayama together, one after the other. Yama and niyama are also very helpful in reducing the rajas and tamas.

Satva is already in me. By reducing the influence of rajas and tamas I will make the satva more and more predominant.

Some people are naturally satvic. For them, the yama and niyama are easy. For instance ahimsa is a characteristic of satva. So, ahimsa becomes easy for them. Others who don't have it naturally will have to practice yama niyama to create an opportunity for satva to come.

But suppose I am a person who is not given to ahimsa. From childhood on I am used to hurting others, physically or by word or thought. This is alright for a normal person because you are dealing with others of similar sentiments. But when you want to take to Yoga you have to come out of this mold. The yamaniyamas will have to be practiced. For those they don't come to naturally it takes special effort to cultivate these habits. Over time, the yamaniyamas together with asana, pranayama, and pratyahara bring the chitta from one which is either tamasic or rajasic to one which is predominantly satvic. Once I become a predominantly satvic person then I am really a yogi. When the mind becomes satvic then I am able to use that satvic mind to understand things which I am not able to understand normally.

A satvic mind is very orderly, dharmic. It does not take anything which does not belong to him. All the yamaniyamas will come under dharma. Ahimsa will come naturally. He will not harm anybody. It will be against his nature to harm anybody. Satya. To speak untruth also is against his nature. Tapas. Clogging the senses with a lot of stimulus is against his nature. All the yamaniyamas become part of his personality. He becomes so satvic that he will be able to contemplate on the spiritual matters that are mentioned in Yoga, Vedanta, etc. Once you are in a satvic mold Yoga comes naturally.

Influence of Outside World

The entire universe is made up of Satva, Rajas, and Tamas. We are being constantly bombarded by rajasic influence and tamasic influence from outside. So, to reduce the rajasic and tamasic influence the yamas and niyamas are very helpful. The yamas and niyamas are a good way to try and reduce the influence of the external world on you. Because if you don't do that, if you try to make your own body and mind satvic without stopping the influences from the outside world then it may not work because it constantly seeps in, as if by osmosis. It gets into your system constantly. The yamaniyamas are a good barricade to see that the outside influence of rajas and tamas don't bother you.

Yamaniyama talks about proper satvic food. Yamaniyama talks about your associations with other people. Yamaniyama talks about the influence of other people on you.

Gunas and the Time of Day

The daytime, between sunrise and sunset is a rajasic period. That's when people go and do their work, in the daytime. From sunset to early morning, before dawn, that is the tamasic time. That is the time when it is better to sleep. But, about an hour and a half before dawn, that is the time when the environment is full of satva. So that is the time for your yoga practice, your meditation, etc.

The more time you spend awake at night the more tamasic you become. Because how we behave during daytime and how we behave during night time are different the influence of time and also the influence of place have an affect on us.

When do I sleep, when do I study, when do I practice. All these are important. All are based on the three gunas. Look for satva. Look for the satvic food. Look for the satvic people around us. Look for satvic practices. Chanting is a satvic practice. It improves us.

Yoga and Sāṁkhya go into the three gunas as no other subject does, so that you will know what to do and what not to do. What to eat and what not to eat. What to study and what not to read. What sort of practice to do and what practices to avoid.

The Gunas and the Four Purushārthas

Human beings have set for themselves four goals: dharma, artha, kama, and moksha.

Dharma is orderliness. There are people who are compassionate, who do their duty completely, do whatever is mentioned in their religion, are law abiding. This is dharma. Their entire life is: I will do my duty according to the law. Such people are satvic.

Artha means possessions, acquisitions. People who try to collect a lot of things. A spouse, a family, a house, property, friends, etc. It grows. They keep on collecting. This is rajasic temperament.

Kama means satisfaction of sensual desires. I want food when I'm hungry. Almost like animals. All the senses have to be kept satisfied. Towards that I will do anything. This is tamasic.

Moksa. People who would like to get released for the previous three. For such people the three gunas are in a state of equilibrium.

Basically, each goal comes form which guna predominates.

To summarize:

The Three Gunas and the Four Human Goals (Purushārthas)

1. People who lead a Dharmic life (life of orderliness and charity) are predominantly Satwic.

2. People who pursue Artha (wealth, possessions and power) are predominantly Rajasic.

3. People who pursue Kama (gratification of senses/ after intense pleasure experiences) are predominantly Tamasic.

4. People who work toward Moksha (ultimate spiritual freedom/ release) tend to overcome the influences of the three Gunas (nistraigunya – as mentioned in the Gita).

3

The First Step: Kriya Yoga

Starting Point

At the start of Chapter II of the YS, Vyasa in his commentary calls those for whom Chapter I is applicable samahita chittas, those whose mind is in a state of samahita. Sama means balance and hita means soothing or peaceful. There is no pain. The mind is not easily disturbed. These are people who are already in a state of peace. They are born yogis -- unlike the rest of us who are constantly in a lot of pain, whose minds are constantly being distracted, constantly going out through the senses.

How do we design a program suitable for people like us? People who are easily distracted, but interested in Yoga? There must, of course, be some interest otherwise there is no point in discussing it.

These people see themselves to be suffering. The suffering is due to basic tendencies of outward movement of the mind. But at the same time they don't have the capabilities to change this movement. For such people the second chapter starts.

What can be done for a mind which is constantly going out through the senses? How can such a mind be made able to achieve the goals of Yoga? First of all this outward tendency or force will have to be curtailed before it can begin the journey in the opposite direction.

Vyasa says that now (after having given instruction for the devotee capable of Samadhi in Chapter I) the instruction begins for how a student with a distracted mind can attain Yoga. Slowly this group of students will be led to the experiences of the first chapter.

Patañjali starts Chapter Two with a simple form of Yoga called Kriya Yoga. Kriya means action. Less thinking and more practice is involved. The mind has been going in a particular direction; it needs to be stopped, and then turned back. He gives a few activities that he suggests will be helpful to begin reversing the movement of the mind. Kriya Yoga, according to Patañjali, consists of three components: tapas, svādhyāya, and iśvara praṇidhānāni.

Tapas

Tapas is a term found in the Vedas. It literally means to heat. The example given is metal. When you heat metal all the dross goes away and the metal becomes purified. This is the way gold is refined. So, tapas here refers to acts of purification. Tapas is certain activities which purify the body, the senses and the mind.

Krishnamacharya. would say that tapas basically involves two activities, moderation of speech and moderation in food. He would also include simple postures.

Don't say anything which is unnecessary. Sometimes you say something and then someone else says something and then you say something in response, and so on. At the end of it you don't feel happy about the whole thing. The mind has grown tired and you said things that you should not have said. A mind gets disturbed from unnecessary talk.

The first thing a yogi has to do is curtail his talk and moderate his food. He can't be a glutton and still want to be a yogi. Many of the texts talk about how much and what kind of food to eat.

We're supposed to eat until the stomach is half full. A quarter of the stomach should be filled with water. The other quarter should be left free for digestion.

Basically, the texts like the HYP, the Gita, and several others say you must curtail rajasic and tamasic food and take satvic food.

What is satvic food? Satvic food is food that does not create tension in the system. Foods that are easily digestible: grains, fruits, milk, veggies. You don't want to eat foods that are too heavy and you don't want to eat too great a quantity. Which is to say, you don't want to overload your disgestion lest you snuff out the agni, the digestive fire.

Rajasic and tamasic food have a tendency to disturb the mind. Tamasic food makes the mind dull. Rajasic food gets the mind excited. Some people say that when they take a lot of sugar their mind gets excited. They can't sleep. It you drink too much coffee in the evening you can't sleep. If you drink certain beverages the mind becomes dull.

Food has an affect on the mind. We all know that. Some foods have an immediate affect; some have a long standing affect. If I'm serious about Yoga I have to take care of my food because the food that we eat becomes part of us. And then part of that becomes my mind and then the mind is going to be disturbed if the wrong food or quantity is eaten.

So, for beginning level yogis, for instance someone who has worked for most of his life and now wants to take care of himself and looks to Yoga so he can have some peace of mind, for such people the first advisory given by Patañjali is: Don't talk too much; Don't eat too much.

Moderation actually refers not only to food, but to everything you take in through the senses. What we hear, what we see, what we smell, what we eat. Sound, news, food, entertainment, etc. The input is all of them put together. I have to pay some attention to this input. Before you go to bed sit down and think: what are the various things you heard during the day. What are the various things that you have done during that particular day. All these things have an affect on the mind. These are the inputs; these are things we have taken through the senses.

This moderation gives free space to the mind and we feel less stressed. This is the vacation effect. We go to Hawaii, we lie on the beach, we don't keep up with the news, we turn off the cell phone, we kick back and the mind relaxes

Tapas means making the necessary effort to see that you don't take rajasic and tamasic inputs from the outside. The more you take rajasic and tamasic food from outside, food for thought, food for all the senses, the more the mind is going to be disturbed. Rajas has a tendency to make your mind agitated. Tamas has the tendency to make the mind dull. I have to avoid taking these types of food and slowly start taking more and more satvic, moderate food. This is the first suggestion. It is very down to earth. We are not talking about Samadhi here.

Svādhyāya

The second component of Kriya Yoga is svādhyāya. Adhyāya = study; svā = self. Some translate this as the study of any subject which sheds light on the self. But classically svādhyāya meant study of the Vedas and chanting of mantras. For the Vedas talk about the true nature of the Self. In fact there is a chapter in the Vedas called svādhyāya prakarana. It deals with Vedic study, especially the Gayatri.

So Svādhyāya refers more or less to all those texts which help you understand your own self. For first of all you must get theoretical knowledge. If I want to become a Yogi I should study Yoga texts. The Yoga Sutra says this, the Hatha Yoga Pradipika says this, the Upanishads say this. We should know these things. For us, it is sufficient to begin study with the YS and Sāṁkhya Kārikā. It is best to study authentic texts.

Iśvara praṇidhāna

The third component is Iśvara praṇidhāna. Here this refers to karma Yoga which means you go about doing your duty without worrying about the results. You do your activity and leave the rest to God. That kind of attitude is called Iśvara praṇidhāna.

Normally we do something and immediately we think about the results. If the results are not to our expectations we worry about it or we are unhappy. But if you want to take up Yoga just go about doing your duty whether you get the results expected or not. Don't worry about it. Regarding the results of activity there should be a mental attitude of surrender to the Lord. If you do that an enormous burden to the mind is removed.

There is another way to understand Iśvara praṇidhāna. That is as iśvara pujana. Here, since we are not capable of meditation yet (because our minds are disturbed), this refers to any kind of worship from your own religion that you are comfortable with. Doing iśvara pujana on a daily basis brings a certain discipline to the mind.

Some say this is more appropriate here and surrender is more appropriate later in aṣṭāṅga yoga.

It is not clear from the text which interpretation of Iśvara praṇidhāna is correct. Both are appropriate and you may do whatever appeals to you.

Summary

We might summarize by saying kriya yoga means eat less, study, and pray.

Or, we might say Kriya Yoga basically refers to Moderation, Study, and Surrender to the Lord.

For a beginning level yogi there is no point in talking about Samadhi, the true nature of the Self, etc. If you start with these things he is going to be more confused. So, Patañjali starts with Kriya Yoga. This is the minimum. The first step is always some kind of restriction on food. Control the intake. Food basically, but, as we have said, it also refers to things we take in through our senses: what we hear, what we see, what we eat, and so on.

Niyama and Kriya Yoga

Later in Chapter II tapas, svādhyāya, and iśvara praṇidhāna occur again as part of Niyama. We take Niyama to include Kriya Yoga.

Benefit

When you practice kriya yoga what is the benefit? It prepares the mind for Samadhi. It does not produce Samadhi, but the mind is prepared for it. It puts you on the right path.

Anyone who starts on kriya yoga is already in a lot of pain. He is not happy. He wants to see if the yoga will make him calmer, more peaceful. Kriya yoga reduces all the causes (the kleśas) that create pain in the mind. The pain he experiences is lessened. It doesn't completely eliminate the pain, but it reduces it substantially.

(YS II.2) The mind becomes fit for samādhi and those attitudes or conditions of the mind which cause pain (kleśa) are greatly reduced.

There are immediate short term benefits. The mind becomes more sattvic, capable of samādhi, and with such a mind we can begin the practice of yoga. And, the mental pain is greatly reduced. Kriya yoga is to reduce pain and suffering by reducing the causes of pain i.e. the kleshas. So, even if one is not interested in the final goal of yoga there are great benefits from kriya yoga. For some, this in itself may be sufficient.

4

The Kleśas

What are the kleśas?

Kleśa = that which causes pain; the colorings of the mind. Kleśa produces duḥkha or pain in us.

Patañjali says (YS II.3) there are five causes of pain: Avidyā asmitā rāga dveṣa abhiniveśāḥ panca kleśāḥ.

Avidyā

Vidyā means knowledge. So avidyā means 'not knowledge', that is 'wrong knowledge'. It does not mean lack of knowledge or ignorance. If I don't know something that is not avidya. I know something, but the knowledge I have is wrong. Misunderstanding. Mistake. That is called avidyā. The knowledge that this particular body is the Self is wrong according to the yogis. It is avidyā.

Asmitā

Asmi mean 'I am'. Asmitā literally is the 'I am' feeling, the 'I exist' feeling. The experience that I exist. That 'I exist' feeling is a klesha. I forget it when I sleep or somebody hits my head. Otherwise this feeling is there all the time. It is wrong knowledge about the Self. This "I" in the "I exist" feeling is not the real Self.

Rāga

Rāga is attachment, to be always in pursuit of objects which are favorable to us. Attachment appears to be pleasure, but it produces its own kind of pain. If the object we are attached to is not available it produces a lot of pain. If I am addicted to coffee, or addicted to something else, and I don't have it I am miserable. So rāga also produces pain.

Dveṣa

Dveṣa is dislike or hatred, avoiding objects which are unfavorable. I hate certain things. Because they have caused me pain before. E.g. If I have arthritis it produces pain. So I want to get rid of it. I take medicines; I go to this doctor, that doctor. If there's somebody I don't like then I want to get away from that person.

Abhiniveśāḥ

Abhiniveśāḥ means fear. Fear of losing what we have: of losing relationships, property, of losing things we're attached to. Fear of losing what we like. Fear of being bothered by what we don't like. I'm always afraid of being harmed by forces that are inimical to me. Because of rāga and dveṣa we have abhiniveśāh, fear.

The height of all these fears is fear of losing the particular person I think I am, the mind-body complex. That is what I am most attached to. That is what I am most afraid of losing. And, when do I lose this? When I die. So the culmination of this fear is the fear of death.

Reduce the Kleśas

These are the five kleshas. Through the practice of kriya yoga the effects of these start to be reduced. There are some people who are so attached (rāga) to other people or things that they could kill. Likewise dveṣa. There are those who could go to any extreme out of hatred. This intense raga, dvesa or intense fear should be reduced. Otherwise it's going to bother us all through our lives.

The Breeding Ground

(YS II.4) Avidyā is the breeding ground for the rest and they can be in any one of four states: dormant; sometimes sprouting, sometimes dormant; sometimes manifest; manifest all the time.

The wrong knowledge that this particular body is the Self leads to asmitā, rāga and dveṣa. Because I called this person "me". That is asmitā. "I exist." "I exist." Where do I exist? In this body. This is wrong knowledge.

Once I am able to identify this body as the Self then I divide all the objects around me into "this I like" and "this I don't like." The objects may include people. The objects may include ideas, thoughts, feelings. I am attached to objects which give me happiness; I am averse to objects which give me unhappiness. Raga and dvesha. It happens because I am identifying this body with the Self.

I am so attached to this particular person. All through my life I have been attached to this particular person. So I am afraid of losing this particular person. That is called abhinivesa.

Eliminate the Root Cause.

Avidyā is wrong knowledge. Basically, it is wrong knowledge about ourselves. It is the breeding ground for the other kleshas. It is the cause of the other kleshas. They all emanate from avidyā. So, there's no point in trying to work on the other four kleshas. Rather, try to work on avidyā itself. Try to reduce avidya. The more you reduce avidyā, the more the others will fall as well.

For some people klesha arises out of raga; for some out of dvesha; for some pain may arise out of fear. The way we experience pain will vary. Some people experience pain because they are attached to everything. That's a big problem. Raga is the main problem for them. On the other hand, there are some people who develop dvesha, they start hating everybody. But both groups feel pain. The same goes for fear. The moment I get a headache I immediately think I have a brain tumor. Whatever the reason they all produce pain. But Patañjali suggests you don't try to sort out each of these problems separately. The root cause of all these is avidyā, your misunderstanding about the nature of your own Self.

Avidyā is of Four Types

We can have Avidya with different groups of objects.

Things which are not permanent, impermanent we consider to be permanent. For example, my own body is not permanent. Yet I keep on doing things as if I am going to live forever. I plan for the next 30 years. We never think of ourselves as impermanent.

Things which are not pure, impure we consider to be pure. The body is unclean. It constantly produces waste products. It constantly requires cleaning. Yet we consider it to be clean. According to Yoga, everything in Prakriti is impure when compared to the purity of the soul.

Sometimes we think what is painful is giving us happiness. Pain is considered to be happiness. It is all part of Prakriti.

We consider the non-Self to be the Self. My mind-body complex is the non-Self but I consider it to be the Self and act as if this is the Self and then try to work out a lot of things to make this wonderful person happy. I keep on doing this. All my efforts are to make this person happy. I've been doing it all my life. I continue to do that.

Each of these is called avidyā. Avidyā is a complete misunderstanding of reality.

The view of Yoga is that all objects are impermanent, not clean, a source of pain and unhappiness, and not the Self. According to Yoga everything is impermanent except the Self. Everything is unclean because of the presence of rajas and tamas. Nothing gives permanent happiness; everything ultimately results in pain. The body-mind complex is non-Self

We attribute permanence, purity, source of happiness, and self to objects. This imposition of wrong ideas is called avidyā.

Kleshas as Five Kinds of Wrong Knowledge

The afflictions (kleshas) can be analyzed as five forms of wrong cognition. They're called afflictions as they are the root causes of misery and impediments to mokṣa.

Avidyā is wrong notion about objective things: mistaking the non-eternal for the eternal, the impure for the pure, the painful for the pleasurable and the non-self for the Self.

Asmitā is wrong notion about subjective things: identifying one's Self with one's body and mind.

These two are intellectual defects.

Rāga and dveṣa are emotional weaknesses.

The sense of permanence in transient things is the chief symptom (of Avidyā) in Abhiniveśa.

In attachment the chief one is a sense of purity in impure things.

Hatred is marked by feeling pleasure in the painful, because though hatred is a form of misery, it appears to be pleasant or desirable. (Hariharananda II.2-5)

Avidyā is the determinant of all feelings and emotions. In Sānkhya thoughts and feelings are not regarded as intrinsically different, for the gunas form the materials of both thoughts and feelings.

That Which Sees and That Which Shows

(YS II.6) Dṛk śakti is the principle that has the power to see, the power to observe, the power to know, the power of experiencing. This is the pure consciousness in us. Only the purusha has that power. Darśana śakti is the principle that shows everything, that gives experience to the purusha. Dṛk śakti is the subject; darśana śakti is the object (there is nothing else). Darśana śakti is the mind. I see only what the mind presents to the Self. I don't see objects directly. I see only the chitta vrittis that the mind presents to Purusha. Only the chitta, the mind, has the power to show everything to the Purusha. Without that there is no experience. For an experience to take place there has to be an observer and there has to be a power to show experience to the Self. The Self does not change. It has one power only, the power to see. It is pure consciousness. It is able to observe, that's all. If nothing is shown to it, it will not see anything. The Purusha inside cannot see anything outside. It can see only the chitta vrittis. That is known as dṛg-darśana sakti.

In our normal experience the chitta produces another focus. That focus is asmitā, "I exist". I am able to feel I exist. That particular feeling is considered to be "I" even though if you analyze it the moment that "I exist" is known it is part of the chitta vritti because there is only one object. The one object is the chitta vritti. In the chitta vritti there is one part which is "me". That is asmitā. But that is not the real Self. My mind is not able to distinguish between these two because it has avidyā.

Through all that is seen I am able to feel that I exist. The individual self is included in darśana śakti. I am not able to distinguish between the śakti that sees and that which is in the seen. When I am not able to see that distinction it is called asmitā. Asmitā is looking at dṛk śakti and darśana śakti as if they are one. Asmitā is confusing that which sees with that which shows. Just as in a dream where we confuse the Self and the dream self. When we sleep the mind does not identify with the body as the self. Instead it creates a dream self. And then creates different kinds of experiences.

Regarding drg sakti and darshana sakti Patañjali uses the word, "eva" which means as though they are one. They are distinctly different, but in our mind they appear to be one and the same, confusing that which sees with that which shows.

Viveka is the ability to distinguish between these two, Self and individual self.

Aviveka is the inability to make the distinction.

Objects Which are Favorable to Us and Objects Which are Unfavorable

Once asmitā is there then we divide objects into two groups: those which give us happiness and those which do not give us happiness. The mind looks around and says these objects are favorable to me because they gave me happiness yesterday. This particular object gave me unhappiness yesterday or four days back or whatever.

So the mind says ok this is the object that is going to give us happiness let us acquire it, let us keep it. When it comes across objects which give unhappiness it says let us avoid these.

Some objects make your mind relaxed. It may be people, it may be physical things, it may be food, it may be so many things.

Coffee gives my happiness. So I have some kind of attachment to coffee because it has been giving me some kind of happiness. You develop attachment to things which give you happiness. Money gives you happiness because you can buy a lot of things with money. So your eyes open wide when you see money. This is rāga. Because agreeable mental space is provided by these objects, you go to those objects.

Likewise certain objects give me duḥkha, disagreeable mental space. It may be pain or depression, whatever it be. The mind develops aversion, hatred towards those things. Which may lead to activity: let me try and destroy it.

We divide objects in the world into agreeable or disagreeable. My activities are to acquire what I like and to avoid what I don't like. That's how we go through our lives. According to Patañjali it is due to avidyā.

(YS II.7) Attachment (rāga) follows the experience of happiness. Attachment comes because the objects gave me agreeable mental space. I get more and more attached to objects which give me happiness.

(YS II.8) Following the experience of pain or unhappiness is dveṣa or dislike or hatred. I started hated some objects because they gave me disagreeable mental space or duhka. I develop more and more hatred towards objects which give me unhappiness.

Duḥkha

Sukha and duḥkha = agreeable and disagreeable mental space. Even though Patañjali talks about sukha and duhka they are not in equal proportion. Duḥkha is predominant. Sukha comes only once in a while.

If somebody comes to us in a great deal of pain we don't start talking about the nature of the Self. We start with kriya yoga. This will help reduce the pain. Then we can move on to root out the underlying cause. It's like taking Tylenol to reduce the symptom. Even just study of the YS produces a certain calmness in the mind. It doesn't eradicate everything. It doesn't make you a yogi. But at least it gives you another way of looking at things. And, if it appeals to you, you realize you're worrying about things you should not be worrying about.

Even the Scholar

The last klesha is the greatest fear we all have, the fear of death. Abhiniveśaḥ literally means "to remain". Remain in one position. I don't want to leave this body. That feeling is called Abhiniveśaḥ. It is found even among the greatest scholars who have spent their entire lifetime thinking about the nature of Self and the nature of non-Self, etc. Even in them this fear of death is deeply rooted (YS II.9).

Study is Only the Starting Point

That is why an intellectual understanding is not sufficient. The intellectual understanding should lead to inferential understanding (anumana) and ultimately to true direct perception. Until the direct perception takes place the abhiniveśaḥ will continue to be there.

Oh, I studied ten different versions of the YS. X says this, Y says this. I have studied all these things. But it does not make much of a difference. From there you have to go to the next step. You have to internalize the whole thing. Then realize this is what it means. I have to personally start experiencing it. Ultimately, I sit down and meditate and I'm able to see the nature of my own

Self. That's the progression. Mere study is not sufficient. Study is a starting point. It should lead to more and more involvement.

Next: Eradicate the Kleshas

Now, after explaining the five kleshas, Patañjali says (YS II.10) they should be completely eradicated. They should be completely rolled back. The kleshas must be destroyed to make the mind fit for Samadhi and eventually lead to nirodha.

The problem is they are subtle. You can only feel them in your mind. You don't know where raga is, but you know its effects. Do we know where raga sits in our mind? No. Dvesha, where does it sit? We don't know. But it manifests. The same with fear, we don't know. But it manifests. Where is fear? Can you look at where fear is? No. They are so subtle.

In YS II.2, Patañjali says the kleshas can be reduced by kriya yoga. But the kleshas are only weakened by kriya yoga. Now, in YS II.10 he talks of the kleshas being destroyed. So, he has now to give the means for this. We will see they are destroyed by viveka.

Patañjali has described the kleshas as the sources of our pain. But he has not suggested we go through and try to eliminate them one by one. Instead he is leading us to astanga yoga which will lead to realizing the true nature of the Self and this will rid us of avidyā, the root of all the kleshas. They all go in one fell swoop. If you can root out avidyā the mind will no longer be involved in the activities it is involved in now.

How

How can it be done? How can the kleshas be destroyed? By deep contemplation the klesha vrittis will be removed. The word Patañjali uses is dhyāna which means to think or meditate and so here refers to antaranga sadhana, the internal practice of ashtanga yoga which we will come to.

So, YS II.10 says the kleshas should be destroyed; YS II.11 states the means. Kriya yoga is not sufficient. kriya yoga does not talk about dhyāna.

5

Duḥkha (Pain)

When Palliatives No Longer Work

Normally, we deal with pain or duḥkha by finding the cause and treating it. When we have stomach pain or a headache by analysis or scans the cause is found and medicine or treatment given. In this way we are able to overcome pain. If there is mental pain other drugs are available. But, as we get older the fear of death grows stronger and this affects the mind in a different way. Here simple palliative methods do not work. There is something deeper at play.

Yoga deals with this deeper aspect. How? What does Yoga have to say about the nature of pain, it's causes and its cure?

Duḥkha

Viveka means the ability to separate. Viveka means if two things are mixed up you are able to separate them. The viveki can tell right from wrong. So, the Viveki is a person who can sit down and analyze. For the viveki all paths (objects) lead to unhappiness.

Most of the time we are unhappy. Even when we are happy there is in undercurrent of unhappiness. There are factors waiting to make us unhappy.

(YS II.15) Unhappiness is produced by three factors, pariṇāma, tāpa, saṁskāra duḥkhas.

Pariṇāma duḥkha

Parināma means change. Objects keep on changing. Nothing remains the same. What appeared to be good at one time now appears not so good. A job, girlfriend, my own body, my face, they all change. One need only look at some old photographs. Because objects change they give you duḥkha. We like certain things at a particular point of time; after some time we don't like that object anymore. Why -- because the object has changed. What appeared to be good now appears to be not so good.

In addition, the mind itself is an object and as such it too changes over time. This may create duḥkha as well. See below under guṇa vṛtti virodhācca.

Tāpa duḥkha

Tāpa is thirst. Tāpa duḥkha is of two types: the inability to get what you want and your inability to get rid of what you don't want.

You may be a good yoga student. You do your practice. You become a teacher. You can explain everything. But still you don't attract many students. Whereas someone else who you consider an upstart, who says things you don't consider to be yoga, in a short period of time comes to be considered a great yogi. So, what do you say? What is it I have not done to be as famous as somebody else? What good deeds have I not done to become like this? That is tāpa. We have this tāpa all the time. All of us have a certain degree of unhappiness due to non-achievement. I might have achieved a lot, but still I compare myself with someone else. There is a difference between expectations and what you've got. Tāpa here means you want something and you are not able to get it. There is restlessness in the mind: I have to solve this problem. That is tāpa.

There is also another tāpa. Look at the other yogi who has become very well known. The same yogi I have been comparing myself to and been unhappy. Look at that particular person. He's got his own problems. He's so famous he can't make any mistakes. He has to be very careful. He has to be on guard all the time. A lot of money is involved. He has to worry about it. If, in addition, he has some ailment he says to himself, what sins have I committed to suffer like this. There is pain there.

There is pain there; there is pain here.

Saṁskāra duḥkha

Saṁskāra means habit. This is duḥkha coming from habits. After 40 years of being a CEO I decide I want to be a yogi. I start, but all the saṁskāras, the way I have conducted my life, they don't change. It takes a very long, dedicated effort to change my saṁskāras my old habits. If I am a smoker, how difficult it is for me to quit smoking. These saṁskāras are in us. My mind is nothing but the remainder of my saṁskāras. Saṁskāra duḥkha is the pain which comes from being unable to change my habits. All my life I have been associating myself with the body-mind complex. I am not able to change this. Why? Because of my saṁskāras.

Guṇa vṛtti virodhācca

I am made up of the three gunas. My mind is made up of the three gunas. What happens? When the gunas change the way I think also changes. When you are in a satvic mold you are so happy. If somebody says something demeaning about you it just rolls off and you forget it. On the other hand, if rajas is dominant the next day, someone may say something which is nothing compared to what was said the previous day, and immediately you lose your temper. And, when tamas dominates again your behavior is different. Constantly we change.

Each of the three guṇas is opposed to the other two. The same person acts or thinks differently depending on the guṇa which dominates. We may act under the influence of one guṇa and regret that action when another guṇa dominates. We may go to a party one night and regret what we did or said the next morning. During the previous night you were in the tamasic mold; on the previous day you were in a rajasic mold, and so on. Depending on which guna dominates at a particular period of time your behavior changes.

So, as the mind changes under the influence of different guṇas, this too gives unhappiness. It produces duḥkha. There is nothing constant or permanent about my own behavior.

To the Viveki All is Pain

So, the yogi, the viveki, who can analyze these things sees parinama duḥkha, saṁskāra duḥkha, tāpa duḥkha, guna vritti duḥkha and concludes from all this it is not worthwhile to constantly try and work towards happiness. It is not there.

For example, there is a lot of pain acquiring wealth. You've got to work hard. For a few it comes easily, but for most of us you've got to work hard. Then to protect that wealth you've got to be careful. You put the money in a particular bank or stock or buy a property. Then the property price goes up or comes down. Then foreclosure happens. Or somebody steals from you. Again there is duḥkha. Then you start using it up. I had a million dollars a few years back. Now it is down to a hundred thousand. We don't feel those things; we keep on working. But for a viveki who sits down and analyzes the question arises: is it worthwhile doing all these things to get a small amount of happiness here and there?

As Vyasa puts it in his commentary on YS II.15, "... a wise man is like an eyeball. Just as a thread of wool which falls on the eyeball gives pain by its touch but not when it falls on other parts of the body, so these miseries affect only a Yogi who is as sensitive as an eyeball and not another who comes in touch with them."

What is the Cause of Duḥkha?

Duḥkha is caused by the mixing up of the Purusha with the projection by the mind of the false self, avidyā.

This time Patañjali comes at the question from a different angle. Instead of saying the cause is that there is no proper knowledge of the Self, Patañjali in YS II.17 says the cause is the mixing up of the Self or the observer and that which is experienced. What is experienced? Chitta vrittis. The cause of duḥkha is the complete mixing up between the Observer and the observed. The observed is the chitta vrittis.

In the chitta vrittis there is a focus about ourselves. In the chitta vrittis there is a feeling of "I exist". The mind identifies with that feeling and continues to operate. So instead of knowing the difference between the Purusha and the observed there is a complete mixup between the Purusha and the observed. The mind is not able to distinguish between Purusha and prakriti, between Purusha and the asmitā feeling. So long as the mind is not able to distinguish it will operate as though this asmitā is the Self and then does everything to satisfy this pseudo self, the wrong self. And that, according to Patañjali, is the cause of all the pain.

6

Aṣṭāṅga Yoga – The Means

The Problem

By kriya yoga the mental pain, duhkha, can be reduced. However, it should be completely eradicated. The duḥkha is to be completely destroyed achieving a state of no pain. By what means can this be accomplished?

(YS II.25) According to Patañjali when avidyā becomes non-existent the mixing up of the Self and the non-self also goes away. And, this mixing up is the cause of duḥkha (YS II.17).

How is avidyā destroyed? This happens when we know the nature of the Self.

As Darkness is Dispelled by Light

Just as darkness is dispelled by light, ignorance is dispelled by knowledge. When right knowledge arrives, wrong knowledge departs. Avidyā is destroyed by Viveka Khyāti.

That is freedom of the purusha. That is the state of no pain. When the avidyā is destroyed, the purusha is free. The purusha, which has previously been required to constantly observe all that goes on in the mind, is ultimately not required to see all the confusion, pain and occasional happiness that go on in the mind. When the avidyā is removed, I am free of this pain and confusion.

The means to achieve this is viveka khyāti, discrimination between the nature of the Self and the non-self. When the mind has the ability to distinguish between the Self and the non-self then I am able to see: this is the Purusha and this is the chitta. I am able to see the distinction between these two. For so long the mind has not had this ability.

Well enough, I understand intellectually that purusha is free, etc., but it doesn't happen to me. Why? It is because of old samskaras. I keep returning to my old ways. Old samskaras can be removed by developing new samskaras.

All in the Mind

One technical note. In (SK 62) we learn that Puruṣa is never bound, nor is he released nor does he migrate. It is Prakṛti that migrates, is bound and is released. The Spirit is never bound; it is the mind that is bound. Bondage and release are merely ascribed to the Puruṣa in the same way that defeat or victory is attributed to the King though, in reality, the soldiers are either defeated or victorious. In reality, both enjoyment and release belong to Prakṛti, yet due to the absence of discrimination of Puruṣa being quite distinct from the Prakṛti, they are attributed to Puruṣa.

The notion of bondage is a construct of our minds. It is not a fact about the Self. We only think it is until we have gained discrimination.

Monkey Mind

(YS II.26) The power of discrimination between the Purusha and the Prakriti, between the Self and the pseudo-self, must be constant in the mind. Viplavā means the continual jumping around of the mind. It keeps on changing, like the activity of a monkey. What does a monkey do? It jumps from one branch to another. And then it jumps to another branch. The monkey keeps on jumping. What we are after is the opposite, aviplavā. The discrimination between Purusha and Prakriti should become your dominant thought. The mind should become steady with this knowledge of the distinction between Prakṛti and Purusha. That is aviplavā. That is the means of destroying the avidyā.

One moment I have the knowledge of the Self. The next moment I have the knowledge of the Self. And, so on. The mind remains steady with that knowledge. There is no point in merely knowing about it just for one moment and forgetting about it the next. That doesn't help. It has to become the dominant chitta vritti in me.

Over a period of time the mind develops this saṃskāra. It is very simple, but very difficult.

Aviplavā – The New Saṃskāra

The next question is how to get this aviplavā, a mind which is constantly watching the distinction between Purusha and Prakriti. Aviplavā vivekakhyāteḥ is the means of destroying avidyā. How do we acquire that?

Put another way, we might ask: I've been doing kriya yoga. I've successfully reduced the kleshas. I'm in a receptive state of mind. Now, how can I make my mind constantly aware of viveka?

For this Patañjali gives a more elaborate procedure: Aṣṭaṅga Yoga.

Aṣṭāṅga Yoga – The Axe

The answer is Aṣṭāṅga Yoga. Vyasa states it this way in his commentary to YS II.28: "Practice of Yogāṅgas is the means of eradicating the impurities as an axe is the means of severing wood."

(YS II.28) All the aspects or limbs (aṅgas) of Yoga have to be practiced. You have to stay in each stage, without wavering, remaining steadfast, practicing correctly and faithfully, completely mastering each limb. Then the impurities, rajas and tamas, are reduced. They become virtually inoperable. Sattva becomes dominant. And, the light of knowledge (about the nature of Purusha and Prakriti) leads to vivekakhyāti, the ability to discern between the Self and the non-self.

A steadfast practice of Aṣṭāṅga Yoga will take the mind to a state where it will be able to see the distinction between Prakriti and Purusha.

How Long Will It Take?

Once I start on the path of Yoga, how long will it take? When will I transform my mind and reach complete freedom? It may happen in this janma (birth) for some people or it may take place after several janmas. It depends on the amount of effort that you put in, the intensity of effort, and where you start from.

Deep Cleaning

With the practice of Kriya Yoga a certain amount of cleaning of the mind takes place, the removal of gross impurities. Now you want to go deeper. The example is given of an earthen pot with lots of pores in it. Suppose you store kerosene in it. Then the smell of kerosene fills all the pores. If you want to clean it you first empty the pot and scrub it inside and out. But, because the pores have been filled up, if you try and store some other liquid, it will still have the strong smell of the kerosene. If you want to be rid of the kerosene completely you normally heat the pot. Then the smell of the kerosene is removed.

Likewise Aṣṭaṅga Yoga is a deeper practice than Kriya Yoga. Kriya Yoga does a certain amount of cleaning. It makes you fit for further Yoga. But it will not take you to vivekakhyāti. For that you must adopt and practice a much more organized form of Yoga, virtually a full time Yoga. Aṣṭaṅga Yoga is a full time Yoga practice.

The Aṅgas (limbs) of Yoga

What are the aṅgas (limbs) of Yoga? The aṅgas are (YS II.29):

1. yama
2. niyama
3. āsana
4. prāṇāyāma
5. pratyāhāra
6. dhāraṇā
7. dhyāna
8. samādhi

Since there are eight aṅgas it is called Aṣṭaṅga Yoga.

Outline

Yama means to control. Yama tells you the yogi's relationship with the outside world. Yama tells you the control (of oneself) one has to exercise with respect to the outside world. What should my relationships be with other beings? What should my relationships be with objects in the outside world? The rules by which the yogi has to conduct himself with respect to the outside world are covered by Yama. Without this guidance you'll be completely distracted by the outside world.

For example, the first yama is ahiṁsa. The yogi's relationship with all other beings is to be governed by the rule of ahiṁsa. It is only for the yogi. It is not for everybody else, not for ordinary people. If you want to be a yogi, if you have decided to follow the path of Astaṅga Yoga then you must practice ahiṁsa without exception. You cannot practice ahiṁsa except when you are angry. It will not work.

Certain personal self-restraints, or habits, are also necessary. Niyama are personal habits one has to develop which are not distracting.

The third aṅga is called āsana. Āsanas are certain physical exercises which keep one in good health. A yogi has to be healthy. The rajo guna is reduced by āsana. The more rajas one has the sicker he becomes. Āsana was the means by which the yogis were able to eradicate disease so they could maintain good health for all the time they were practicing Yoga. Through a regular practice of āsana the yogis developed a system by which they were able to maintain good health all through their lives.

This is one meaning of āsana, postures for health. There is another. Literally āsana means seat. So āsana means how you sit. Specifically, a classical seated position which you can stay in for a long period of time. This is necessary because classically it was said that for meditation you need to be able to sit comfortably for a long time. Meditation is not done while you are moving. The whole purpose of āsana is to be able to stay, keeping the body steady, for a long period of time without any aches and pains.

Then comes Prānāyāma, control of breathing. If the breathing is not properly controlled yogis found the mind cannot be controlled. So they want to use prāṇāyāma to control the mind. Mere asana practice is not sufficient. Prānāyāma removes the tamo guna from the system.

The next aṅga is called pratyāhāra. Having done āsana and prānāyāma, pratyāhāra becomes necessary. Why? Because you don't want the senses to distract you now. You've taken a lot of effort, you've reduced your rajas and tamas and now your mind, which is satvic, is capable of meditation. To allow the senses to again distract the mind is not going to be helpful. So I must do a specific practice so the senses are also brought under control. Such a procedure is called pratyāhāra. Stop the activity of the senses, at least for a short period of time. Close the eyes, close the ears, go to a place where there is not much distraction. Then the senses will not automatically drag you outside.

With yama you have developed a cordial relationship with the outside world. With niyama you have developed certain personal habits which are not distracting. Then you practice āsana so you have a better control over your body. You practice prānāyāma so you have better control over your mind. You did pratyāhāra so you have better control over your senses. Having done all these practices now you are prepared for meditation.

These first five aṅgas are called baharaṅga sādhana. Anybody can see and judge your practice of these. A teacher can tell if you are doing these practices correctly. The next three are called antaraṅga sādhana. This is an interior practice, a practice for the mind. Only you can know if you are making progress here.

Patañjali divides meditation into three stages. The first stage is called, dhāranā; the second stage is called, dhyāna; and the third stage is called, samādhi. Unless you are able to do dhāraṇā you will not be able to do dhyāna; unless you are able to do dhyāna you will not be able to do samadhi. Each one leads to the next.

A Complete System

Patañjali has presented, in Aṣṭanga Yoga, a very systematic method. Each one of the aṅgas has a reason why it is there. To reach the goal one has to master all the limbs. They are all necessary.

Yama is necessary because I am living in this world. Niyama is necessary because as a being my body and mind have certain tendencies. I have to bring them under control. I have to develop a good, healthy physical body. So, I've got to practice exercises. What exercises are most suitable for a yogi? They are āsanas. Then I've got to do prāṇāyāma. I need breathing exercises. Breathing exercises help you to clear the mind. You also have to control the senses, hence pratyāhāra. It's a very nicely developed system. Once you practice the first five aṅgas your mind will be in a better condition to go into meditation. For that, the next three aṅgas are there. You can't take shortcuts with the system. You can't say, "Oh, I just meditate. I don't do āsanas, I just go straight into meditation." It doesn't work.

7

Yama Niyama

Yamas

The five yamas (restraints or controls) are: ahiṁsa, satya, asteya, bramhacarya, aparigraha.

Ahiṁsa

Ahiṁsa means nonviolence. Hiṁsa is to harm (any being); ahiṁsa is to not harm. Of all the dharmas or virtues ahiṁsa is the highest. Ahiṁsa refers to all the beings outside us. Your relationship with all the beings outside you should be governed by the principle of ahiṁsa. The yogi should not harm anybody. The reason you should not harm anybody, in practical terms, is because if you harm somebody they are going to come back at you.

You can hurt somebody by deeds, by words, and by thoughts. Some people physically hurt others; some people verbally hurt others; some people mentally have negative thoughts about other people. All these, whether they hurt other people or not, are going to hurt the yogi himself. That is why he has to practice ahiṁsa.

You should not physically harm somebody. If you have to say something you should say it in such a way that it will not hurt. You should not think of harming somebody.

Unless you are becoming a yogi ahiṁsa cannot really be practiced because there is a certain amount of violence inherent in everyday activities such as killing of mosquitoes, etc.

Hiṁsa is without beginning, but it can end.

Satya

Satya means speaking the truth. Satya is truthfulness in communication. I must communicate only what is true.

Ahiṁsa may also refer to communication. Sometimes speaking the truth might harm somebody. These are conflicting dharmas (virtues). One dharma is to speak the truth; the other dharma is not to harm anyone. Never say something which is true which is going to cause harm to other people. What you say should be true and it should create good will. Keep this in mind all the time.

It is a difficult situation, but you have to develop a way to say what is true and create good will.

You don't have to say everything that is true. Even though it is true, you can observe silence. Conversely, even though it may be pleasing to somebody you should not say something that is false. If you are a music teacher with a terrible student you should not tell her mother how beautiful her daughter's voice is just to please her.

Asteya

Steya means to steal. Asteya means to not steal. We should not take things that do not belong to us.

Brahmacarya

The literal meaning of Brahmacarya is a student, one who is studying the Vedas. In the olden days, during the student life, celibacy was maintained. And so, Brahmacarya became synonymous with celibacy. But, according to Krishnamacharya, for the householder Brahmacarya means not transgressing the institution of marriage.

Aparigraha

Aparigraha means non-accumulation, not to accumulate. Parigraha is to accumulate, to keep on taking and collecting. But once you accumulate things you have to take care of them. The more houses you own the more problems you have managing them. It is going to distract you from the path of Yoga, taking you in a different direction.

Aparigraha means you take only what is necessary. Anything beyond what you need you don't try to accumulate. Aparigraha is for the Yogi. It is not for the businessman. It is not for people in the yoga business. The one who desires to be a Yogi should have minimum belongings.

A Story

Once there was a yogi living a few miles away from a village. After some time he got a student who wanted to become a yogi himself. The student came and stayed with the yogi and the yogi began teaching him āsana, prāṇāyāma, and so on. Then, after some time, he said to his student, I have to go to the Himalayas to do my own tapas. So he left leaving the student to fend for himself.

In the olden days the yogi did not have a home. He would live in a forest or a cave or something like that. And, every day or two he would go to the nearby village and beg for food. The Sannyāsi would go to three houses. He should not take more than one handful of food from a house. He would eat the one handful of food and then go to another house and get another handful and eat. He would eat three handfuls maximum. And, then go back to where he lived.

So, this student, whenever he was hungry, would go to the village and beg for food. Then there came a time when he went and asked in addition for a small piece of cloth. From then on he would receive some food and a small piece of cloth and he would leave.

One day one of the women who gave him alms came out of her house and asked him, "Why do you want this piece of cloth? You ask for it often these days. What's the problem?" He felt shy, but he explained, "The cave where I live is full of rats." As a yogi he was just wearing a loincloth. Every day he would wash and dry it. But the rats would come and destroy the cloth. So, he had to get a fresh piece of cloth. Then the woman asked, "Why do you want to do all that. Why not get a cat? In fact, I have a cat that gave birth to a number of kittens. I'll give you one. You take it and this will take care of the rats and you won't have to worry about them." So, he took the cat. And, the cat ate the rats. And, the student no longer had a rodent problem.

Over a period of time, he came to like the cat. It was a good pet. But it turned out the cat could not exist by eating only rodents. It required milk. So, the next time the student went to the village he did not ask for a piece of cloth, but instead asked for a cup of milk. Every now and then he would ask for a cup of milk. And, they would give it to you.

Then one day another lady asked, "Why do you ask for a cup of milk? You used to ask only for food and now you're asking for milk, too." He explained, "You know, I have to feed the cat I have." So, she gave him the milk. In a few days when he came back again she said, "I have a suggestion. I have two extra cows in my house. I'll give you a cow for the milk." So, he took the cow.

For a few days there was no problem. But – you have to feed the cow. This was not a big problem because he was living in a forest and he could cut some grass. But the cow needed to be cleaned and cared for as well as fed. The disciple did not have the time as he would often sit and meditate and so could not give enough care and attention to the cow. The cow became weak and famished.

The disciple grew worried. When he next went to the village for alms one of the women said, "You look depressed. You don't look like a yogi." He told her the problem was he had to take care of the cow, but did not have the time. This was the same woman who had earlier given him a cat. She said, "You know, I have eight daughters. Why don't you take one of my daughters and marry her? She is very nice and she will take care of the cow." The student said yes and over a period of time they got married and had two children.

Now he spent most of his time taking care of the children, getting food for his family, and so on. For the needs of his family he built a small house in the forest. The disciple was becoming a householder. He got more cows and all that. He started working part time. Now he was just another villager.

Some time after that the senior yogi returned. He had attained his kaivalya and was walking by and saw his disciple in a different lifestyle. The yogi asked his disciple what happened. The disciple narrated the whole story. How it started with the loincloth and so on.

Then the yogi said the solution to the loincloth problem was not to get a cat, but to get rid of the loincloth. Aparigraha.

The Great Vow

These yamas should be practiced by the Yogi all the time, without exception. (YS II.31) This should be observed as a mahāvratam̐ (great vow) by the yogi. This great vow should never be broken. It should not be violated. There should be no exception either for jāti (species), deśa (place), kāla (time), or samaya (occasions). The vow must be kept sārvabhaumāḥ (under all circumstances).

Ok, I will practice ahiṁsā with my children, but not with my neighbor's children. This is exception for jāti. In India people will not harm a cow, but don't mind killing a goat or a pig. This is exception for jāti. Here Patañjali is saying there should be no exception if you want to be a yogi. You should not be cruel to any animal, or any being for that matter. The great vow must be kept regardless of species. There are not certain species which are exempt. This is the meaning of jāti.

Deśa means place. If you go to a temple you practice ahiṁsā. In the temple you're on your best behavior. You don't harm anybody, you don't say anything hurtful. But then when you get out, in different situations, you are a different person. Or, you may feel you would never harm one of your countrymen, but harming people in another country is all right. These are exceptions for deśa. But, by the mahāvrata there is no exception with respect to the place.

Certain people in India won't eat meat during November-December. This is exception for kāla. It is not permitted in the sutra.

Whenever things are fine I am a fine person. When things go wrong I show my true colors. No, samaya means on all occasions.

The mahāvrata is without any exceptions with regard to species, place, time, or occasion. The yogi takes this vow: I will never harm any person. I will never harm any being. I will never say anything false. I will never steal on any occasion. I will maintain brahmacharya on all occasions. I will not accumulate things.

Dharma

There may be an exception because of conflicting dharmas. This was the case for ahiṁsa and satya. It may happen here as well. For instance, if the harming of one may save a hundred then it may be the right thing to do. But, generally the yogi does not find himself in this situation. He has renounced everything. And, for him this becomes a mahāvrata, a great vow.

Kali Yuga

Krishnamacharya once said that in kali yuga the only yama to be practiced is brahmacarya. The rest are very difficult to practice. You have to have money, and so on.

Daily Review

One of the things many of the practical yogis suggest is this: once you decide you want to follow the path of Yoga totally in life then the Yama Niyamas will have to be scrupulously followed. So, every night when you go to bed just have a quick review of what you have done during the day's activities. Ahiṁsa, have I harmed anybody by word, deed, or thought? Satya, did I say anything untrue, knowingly or unknowingly? Asteya, did I take someone else's property? Or, did I take credit for something I have not done? And, so on. There are many ways we can take advantage of someone else's position. Bramhacarya is obvious. Aparigrahā, did I go to work merely to accumulate wealth, etc.?

So, at the end of the day you review these things. You make a conscious effort to review these on a daily basis. Over a period of time the mind changes. You become less violent. You speak less and less untruth. Because these are all habits. Violence is a habit. I used to be a violent person when I was young. So, violence has become a habit. Some people lose their temper easily; some are hard to provoke. If you are used to telling lies when you are young, if it was a childhood habit then, even without your own knowledge, when you speak you start with a lie. Stealing also could be a habit. The same with brahmacharya and aparigrahā.

These are habits one has to overcome. And, a certain amount of effort is required. Patañjali wants the yogi to try and consciously overcome these tendencies.

Niyamas

The next aṅga is called niyama. These are more personal practices. Niyama means to permanently control, all the time. "Ni" refers to a constancy. Everyone will have to do these daily.

The niyamas are śauca (cleanliness), santoṣa (contentment), tapaḥ (control of the senses), svādhaya (study), isvara praṇidhānā (surrendering to the Lord).

Śauca

Śauca means cleanliness. Kkrishnamacharya used to say you should shower before your yoga class. You have to be clean before you start your yoga practice. If you shower first you have a different feeling when you practice yoga than you do if you practice first and shower later on.

Śauca is of two kinds: cleanliness of the body and cleanliness of the mind. The mind normally has lots of thoughts which are not clean. The yogi develops a tendency to ward off the thoughts which are not clean. He has to keep his mind clean as well as his body.

Santosa

Santoṣa means to remain satisfied. It means completely satisfied. Santoasa is to be contented, to keep your mind happy, all the time.

Everyone is in a different situation. Even the same person is in different situations at different times. Some are rich; some are poor. Some are successful; some are not so successful. Some are happy with their family; some are not happy with their family. There are many differences. But the yogi is supposed to remain content in whatever situation he or she is in.

If you crave many things you will not be happy. You will not have a state of mind in which you are content with your situation at any particular moment.
So there are two kinds of tāpas one should not have: why is it I am not like somebody else? And, why am I suffering, what bad deeds did I do to suffer like this?

The idea is: I am in the position I am in because of my own karmas. Nobody else is responsible for that. I can't hold anyone else responsible for the situation I am in. There's no point in blaming anyone else. There's no point in blaming God. There is no point in blaming your parents. Because of my karma I was born to these particular parents. Every one of us is in his/her particular position because of past karmas. So I am responsible for what I am now.

It is not that we should be satisfied it is that we should accept: I am like this because of my own past.

Kriya Yoga

The next three of the niyamas: tapas, svādhyaya, and īsvara praṇidhānāni we have already come across in kriya yoga.

Tapas

Tapas means to keep your senses under control. It means complete control of the senses. According to Krishnamacharya it is moderation in food and moderation in speech.

Svādhyaya

Svādhyaya refers to study of the various texts. Here it refers to study of the Vedas, the scriptures. It can also mean study of those texts which talk about the Self such as the Upaniṣads, Sāṁkhya Kārikā, and the Yoga Sutra.

If you want to be a yogi you have to start studying the theory of yoga.

Isvara praṇidhāna

Isvara praṇidhāna here means surrendering the fruits of karma yoga, the fruits of your actions, to the Lord. Do your yoga practice and at the end make an offering: I have done all this, may I offer the fruits of my actions to you Lord. Surrender yourself to the Lord.

(This is the third time īsvara praṇidhāna is mentioned in the YS. In the first chapter pranava japa is considered īsvara praṇidhāna. In the beginning of the second chapter, in kriya yoga, īsvara praṇidhāna was either puja, the ritual or worship of the Lord, or surrendering the results of your actlons to the Lord.)

Only for the Yogi

These are the niyamas. As is true of the Yamas, these niyamas are only for the Yogi. They are not for all other people. If you want to be a Yogi you have to practice these ten Yama Niyamas. This is called Yoga Dharma. Dharma for the Yogi.

The Problem

So, the yama-niyamas have been mentioned, but because of our old samskaras, because we are not used to these things, we tend to slip back to our old habits.

I have started Yoga, but after some time ... It is like a New Year's resolution. Ok, I am going to practice Yoga. What is the first step? Yama Niyama. Ok, I am going to practice Yama Niyama. What is the first Yama? Ahiṁsa. Ok, I am going to practice ahiṁsa. Then after five minutes my wife asks me something and I lose my temper because I'm used to it. I am not able to maintain ahiṁsa for a long period of time.

So, Patañjali says you have to make a conscious effort to make ahiṁsa part of your psyche. For that, he suggests:

The Solution -- Pratipakṣa Bhāvanaṁ

Vitarka means the opposite, the opposite of all those yama niyamas. What is the opposite of ahiṁsa? Hiṁsa. I have decided to become a non-violent person, but within a short period of time I tend to become violent. So, what is happening? The vitarka is happening. Whatever should not happen is happening. Instead of being a non-violent person I behave as a violent person. That is called vitarka.

If I am affected by the opposite of the yama niyamas, e.g. if I become violent or I start telling lies left and right or I start taking things which don't belong to me or I violate the sanctity of my marriage or I start accumulating – these are transgressions of the vows I've already taken.

For my vow to follow yama niyama not to become just another "New Year's resolution" Patañjali says when you are affected by the contrary tendencies think about the consequences of doing the opposite of yama niyama, pratipakṣa bhāvanaṁ. Pratipakṣa means opposite. Think on the opposite; Reflect on the consequences. What are the consequences of your doing the opposite of your vow?

Consequences

Why did I decide to practice ahiṁsa and the rest? I thought about it. Nobody takes to a serious kind of yoga lightly. I have seen the other kind of life. I know what it is, now I want to try Yoga. That's what I thought. I want to become a Yogi, completely, for the rest of my life.

I start with the yama niyamas. Having started this, when I'm afflicted by the contrary tendencies Patañjali advises: pratipakṣa bhāvanaṁ -- think of the opposite. Reflect on the consequences of the opposite. The opposite of yama niyama means a return to my old way of life, a return to duḥkha.

It's like the vow some people make to give up smoking. If they break this vow, if they begin smoking again, they need to think of the consequences of this.

When your mind tends to the old habits, when you're affected by the old tendencies, you need to realize you're doing the opposite of what you set out to do. You need to think about the consequences of this behavior. This is what it means to think of the opposite.

If I persist with this it is going to produce pain in the future. I was already a person with a lot of pain – that is why I took to Yoga. If I break the vow then I'm going back to the old way of life and the old way of life was painful to me to start with. The old way will produce duḥkha and lack of knowledge (ajñāna) about the Self. I will be in the old groove. That is how you must think of the opposite.

If you do that over a period of time it will help you to go along the path a yama and niyama.

Talk to Yourself

Otherwise the mind cannot be changed. There has to be a conscious effort.

At the end of each day review you behavior with regard to yamaniyama.

Then Patañjali says talk to yourself. Many times when we do something wrong we talk to ourselves. I shouldn't have done this. I shouldn't have done that. We keep on telling ourselves after we make a mistake. The same applies to the practice of yama niyama.

Shame

In Vyasa's commentary he uses a very strong analogy. He gives the example of dogs. Dogs have a tendency to eat their own vomit. If you take to yoga and then start breaking your vows, Vyasa says you are no better than a dog that eats his own vomit.

Vyasa gives this example to create an aversion. He says think of a dog that eats his own vomit. I have vomited this particular way of life. I have thrown it out. I have said I don't want to do hiṁsa because it's not doing me any good. I take the vow of ahiṁsa. Now if I go back to living in the same way as before I am no different than a dog that eats his own vomit.

So you shame yourself. If you violate your vow you say, No, no, what I have done is absolutely unacceptable.

Contrary Tendencies

What are the contrary tendencies? Patañjali explains these next (YS II.34).

Harming, speaking untruth, stealing, opposite of bramhacarya, starting to accumulate wealth. Hiṁsa, asatya, steya, abramhacarya, parigraha. These are the opposite tendencies.

Of Three Types

Hiṁsa and the rest are of three types: I can directly harm somebody, I can ask somebody else to do it, or I can feel vicarious pleasure i.e. if someone else suffers you have a feeling of yes he deserves that, a sense of happiness at the suffering of another.

These are the different levels or ways in which hiṁsa and the rest can happen. I do it myself. For instance, suppose I'm angry with somebody, suppose I'm having an altercation with my neighbor, I go straight away and talk to him and then within a short period of time I lose my temper and I hit him. This is kṛta. I directly do it. I directly become a violent person.

If I am more sophisticated I don't directly go and beat him. I use a hit man. I don't do it myself. I make somebody else do this job for me. I pay him. I sit down and then watch what's going on.

The third possibility is still worse. I don't have the guts to do it myself nor do I have the guts to employ somebody because sometimes these things backfire. If somebody finds out the consequences for me are going to be bad. So, I can't do anything. I keep on wishing ill luck for my neighbor. When something goes wrong for my neighbor, oh yes, I am happy. This is the third kind of violence.

So, Patañjali says be watchful. You sometimes harm others directly, you harm others through some other person, or you feel happy if something goes wrong for them. This last is a very important tendency. Maybe it is a tendency for everybody. When there is pain for somebody, if it is going to produce some kind of happiness in me I should be very careful about that. In German there is a word for this. The word is schadenfreude. Schadenfreude means to feel glee at another's misfortune. This is anumoditāḥ.

When these tendencies arise in me then I must think like this: Oh, these are the tendencies which I wanted to eschew. I didn't want these tendencies to be in me. I may have had it before, but I want to make a conscious decision by which these tendencies, which are basically rajasic and tamasic, will go away from me.

Why They Happen

The reason why I behave like this is because of greed, enmity, or infatuation. Lobha, krodha, and moha; greed, enmity, or infatuation are the reasons why I break my vows. Because of greed I start stealing. Because of krodha I cause harm to other people. Because of moha, infatuation, I break the bramhacharya vow.

Why is it I'm behaving like this? It is because of greed, because of anger or enmity, because of infatuation. These are the factors that force me to break my vows.

Every time I show tendencies of hiṁsa and all that I have to think, ok, these tendencies I find are due to lobha, krodha, or moha. These are the reasons why I have behaved this way. And, if I persist with this I'm going to have endless duḥkha and ajñāna. I will continue to remain in pain and without spiritual knowledge. I'll continue to spend the rest of my life this way. I have to remind myself of this.

Three Grades

These can be of three grades: mild, moderate, or very violent. These will lead to pain and ignorance, and will be without end. In this way, you've got to keep on thinking of the consequences of the opposite.

When I say, no, I am not that violent. It doesn't matter. Violence may be mild or moderate or intense. They are all hiṁsa. You may not be a murderer, but that does not mean you are following the vow of ahiṁsa. Even though your violence is mild it is still hiṁsa.

Number of Sutras

Look at the number of sutras Patañjali has taken to explain yama niyamas. Patañjali discusses yama niyama from sutra II.29 to II.45. Almost 18 sutras are used for yama niyama whereas for asanas he has taken only three sutras.

Stay the Course

So YS II.33,34 give the practical means for how to stay the course with yama niyama.

8

Āsana

Third Anga

Now the third aṅga, āsana.

Three Sutras

Patañjali says everything he has to say about āsana in three sutras. In the first he gives the definition of āsana. In the second he gives the practical methods by which one can achieve āsana siddhi. And, in the third he gives the benefits of āsana.

Definition

What is āsana? The definition is given in YS II.46: Āsana is a yogic posture with two parameters, sthira and sukha, steadiness and comfort. A yogic posture in which one is steady and comfortable is called āsana.

Two Parameters

Patañjali doesn't say āsana means stand on your head or do padmasana. None of those things. He just gives two important parameters so far as āsanas are concerned. Every āsana that you do, you must be steady in it. If there is a posture where you cannot be steady, that is not a yogic posture. Every time you do a posture you must feel comfortable in that. The purpose of āsana is not to make you experience pain. It is to make you experience comfort. That is why they have been chosen. Vajrasana is a lot more comfortable than sitting on a sofa. This is because on a sofa it is unsteady whereas when you sit in vajrasana or padmasana it is steady.

Steadiness and comfort are the hallmarks of a yogic posture.

Of course, you can't be steady and comfortable in a posture the first time. You have to practice regularly. Once you are able to master the posture, that posture will give you a lot of sukha. You can remain in that posture for a long time. There are people who can remain seated in Vajrasana or Padmasana for a very long period of time whereas it is difficult for us to sit on a sofa for a long period of time. Very quickly you have to shift your position. And, you keep on changing.

It is for this reason that the yogis went about developing certain postures they could remain seated in for an extended period of time.

Āsana Means Seated Posture

Why do you want to remain seated for a long period of time? Because you need to stay in a steady, comfortable posture to do Yoga. You need to be steady if you want to do prāṇāyāma. You need to be steady if you want to meditate. Only in a seated posture can you remain steady for a long period of time.

To go into samādhi the yogis had to find postures they could sit in for a very, very long time. They had to come up with postures where the balance would be good. According to them, postures like vajrāsana, siddhāsana, padmāsana, and so on solved the problem.

You can't meditate with a body which is unsteady. So, the reason why āsana is mentioned here is everybody should develop a steady posture. I must physically be steady before I can start thinking of making my mind steady.

There are a number of commentaries, including Sankara's, which suggest that meditation should be done only in a seated posture. The old texts all talk about sitting postures for meditation. You are not supposed to meditate standing. So sthirasukhaṁ āsanaṁ refers to a seated posture.

Standing and Other Āsanas

Conventionally, āsana always refers to a seated posture. Tadāsana, Trikonāsana, etc. are all good, but ultimately I should be able to remain in a seated posture and do prānāyāma and meditation. In śavāsana you can relax, but śavāsana is not a posture for meditation. Stirasukhamāsanaṁ refers ultimately to a seated posture in which you can sit for a long period of time comfortably so that you can meditate.

Later on, when yogis started standing and doing other postures, they also were referred to as āsana. And, they too have to meet the requirements of sthira and sukha. When we teach Virabhadrāsana, etc. we aim for sthira and sukha in the posture. When we stand in Tadasana this is what we look for. This idea of sthira and sukha we can extend to all the yogic postures.

What are the practices that will be helpful for you to achieve perfection in āsana?

Prayatna Śaithilya

"Prayatna Śaithilya" is usually translated as "effortless". But YS II.47 is interpreted differently by different people. Krishnamacharya interprets the sutra saying it is the breath that should be made smooth and effortless.

For us, it should be read along with the previous sutra. Prayatna = effort; śaithilya = to make it light; samāpatti = to focus your attention on. Samāpatti refers to a mental activity; prayatna to a physical activity.

Prayatna is effort. If we refer to the sibling philosophies like Nyāya we find they classify prayatna as of three kinds. All of our activities are divided into three categories: effort to get what you want; activities you do to get rid of something; effort to maintain life. My brain has these three activities. It makes me do things so I can get what I want; it makes me do things so I can get rid of what I don't want. The third effort of my brain is to maintain my life, keep me going. It makes my heart beat, it makes me breathe continuously. It does so many things without my own knowledge.

According to Krishnamacharya, this last, which refers to breathing, is what is meant by prayatna in YS II.47. The technical meaning from Nyāya for prayatna is jivana prayatna or effort toward life i.e. breath. So prayatna should be interpreted as the breath. Then śaithilya is to make it smooth, to make it effortless. If you make your breath smooth and long and not labored – then it is called prayatna śaithilya.

When you practice āsana the breath should be smooth and long, effortless and light.

Focus on the Breath

Many translators say ananta means infinity. You focus your attention on infinity. If you do that and practice āsanas you will get the āsana siddhi. But it is not practical to try and focus on infinity.

Ananta could also mean the original form of Patañjali. But it is unlikely that the author is suggesting meditation on himself.

There is another interpretation of the word ananta. The third meaning comes from "ana" which means to breathe. Ana means breath. For example, prāṇa, apāna, vyāna, and so on. They all come from the root ana, to breathe. So, here ananta refers to breath. Ananta

Samāpatti is to focus your attention on the breath. Anantasamāpatti is to focus your attention on the life force which is breath.

Long Smoothing Breathing with Attention on the Breath

Your breath should be made smooth and long as per the first half of the sutra. And, your mind should be with the breath so far as the second part of the sutra is concerned. We have to have very smooth breathing and our focus should be on the breath. According to Krishnamacharya you will be able to get sthira and sukha in āsana if you practice the āsana with long, smooth inhalation and exhalation and focusing your attention on the breath. If you practice like this then āsana siddhi takes place. You are able to get to the posture correctly within a short period of time.

In āsana practice there has to be a way to make the body relax. That can be done by breathing. So YS II.47 is interpreted as pertaining to the breath. And, along with YS II.46 defines how the āsana practice should be done.

II.46 defines asana; II.47 says how to achieve asana; II.48 gives the benefits.

Benefits of Āsana Practice

From the practice of āsana according to these principles – which leads to mastery -- one is not affected by the pairs of opposites.

Dvandva is the pairs of opposites. A pair of opposites means there are two, but they are in opposite direction. When I am opposing somebody, and there are two people, e.g. if I am having a wrestling match, then it is called dvandva. There are two people, each one fighting the other. On the other hand, if I have a friend it is not called dvandva.

What are the pairs of opposites? Suhka and duḥkha, comfort and pain, they are opposites. Cold and hot, these are opposite. Elation on hearing praise; depression on being criticized.

Abhighāta means drowned. Anabhighāta is not drowned or not overpowered. Abhighātaḥ means to be submerged; anabhighātaḥ means he will not be submerged. That is, he won't be overcome. He will not be overpowered. He will not be overpowered by the pairs of opposites.

For instance, suppose I am in a room and the temperature is 70 degrees. This is considered to be a very comfortable temperature. If it goes to 65 degrees I need a heater; if it goes to 75 degrees I need an air conditioner. The range is so small. I'm intolerant. With just a small change I say, oh, come on, let me have a heater. On the other hand, there are people who if it is 50 degrees or 40 degrees they don't complain; if it goes to a hundred degrees they don't complain. They remain unaffected by this.

That is physical, but intolerance can be psychological as well. If somebody says, oh, you are a wonderful teacher, you feel elated. The next moment he says you are lousy, what happens? You go through the floor.

These are the pairs of opposites, praise and ridicule, heat and cold. Being buffeted about by these is intolerance. By regular practice of āsana you become more and more tolerant. You are not easily affected by the pairs of opposites.

That intolerance is said to be a manifestation of rajo guna. Rajas is the quality which makes us intolerant. People who are rajasic are fickled. They have a very short fuse.

When our tolerance limit is exceeded we get angry. The intolerance is a manifestation of the rajo guna. When our tolerance range is very narrow we are affected by the pairs of opposites. So, Patañjali says, by the regular practice of āsana the rajo guna comes down. This is what the commentator of the HYP says as well.

From practicing āsana we become more and more tolerant, i.e. less and less rajasic. The practice of āsana puts us on the path to overcoming the pairs of opposites. Mastery of āsana, the ultimate result of practice, means we have arrived at the goal. We are no longer affected by the pairs of opposites.

Then, once you have reduced the rajo guna a consistent practice is necessary to keep it under control.

The Result

What it means is he will be able to stay in a posture for a long period of time.

9

Prānāyāma

Five Sutras

Patañjali takes a little more time with Prānāyāma than with Āsana. So everybody should do prānāyāma more than āsana. These are the five sutras for Prānāyāma: YS II.49, 50, 51, 52, 53. There are only three sutras for Āsana.

Āsana Siddhi

Sati means remaining; tasmin means in an āsana. Āsana siddhi or mastering āsana means the ability to remain seated in a posture for a long period of time without any discomfort. One should be able to find a posture you can stay in for a long period of time. The sutra (II.49) says first of all we must master an āsana, one posture. Just as people have a favorite mantra, yogis also have a favorite āsana. Classic examples are siddhāsana, vajrāsana, virāsana, padmāsana, gomukhāsana. These are some of the well known seated postures.

Definition

Sutra II.49 defines what prāṇāyāma is. Gati means movement; vicchedaḥ is stopping or interfering with or cutting. Normal breathing is inhalation and exhalation whereas if you deliberately interfere with the breath that is called prānāyāma. Tasmin sati, remaining in a posture such as Vajrāsana, when the movement of inhalation exhalation is cut in various ways, i.e. if you try to stop your inhalation exhalation, it is known as prānāyāma.

Remaining in the asana, breaking or controlling the inhalation-exhalation movement is called prāṇāyāma. If you can deliberately control the inhalation and exhalation then it is called prāṇāyāma. Normally the breathing is not under our control. It takes place automatically. It takes it own course. The yogi controls the inhalation, controls the exhalation, controls the gati, the breath's movement. When he does that, that activity is called prāṇāyāma. When the movement is controlled then it is called prāṇāyāma.

Literally, prāna refers to breathing, āyama is to control. Āyama also means lengthening. So not only must you control the breathing you must lengthen the inhalation and exhalation i.e. you must be able to hold the breath for a long period of time, both in and out. Tasmin sati means you've got to sit in a proper yogic posture to do this.

Meaning

What does it mean? It means you must be able to bring your breathing under your control. Stop anywhere you want. Stop for any length of time you want. That is called viccheda. Cheda is to cut. Viccheda is to cut in different ways. You are able to control the breath, stop the breath in so many different ways. This is called prānāyāma. There's a deliberate attempt to control the breath while remaining in a classical seated posture which you should have mastered so you can stay for a long time.

Teacher

How do we control the breathing? The sutra doesn't tell you how to do that. You must learn this from a teacher and/or other texts. The same is true for āsana. At the same time, other texts like HYP do not give the parameters of āsana that are given in the YS.

Parameters

What are the basic parameters that govern different types of prānāyāma practice? Having defined prāṇāyāma, in the next sutra (II.50) Patañjali gives the factors that should be considered in its practice. All the factors we have to consider in the practice of prāṇāyāma are contained in this particular sutra. What are these parameters? They are: exhalation, inhalation, breath holding, deśa, kāla, saṅkhya, dirgha, and sukṣma. Patañjali tells us all we need to know about prāṇāyāma in one sutra. (He does not mention ujjayi, nadi shodana, etc. These one can find in the HYP.)

Breath Activities (vṛttis)

Vritti here refers to prāna vritti, the activity of the breath. There are three prāna vrittis: bāhya vritti; ābhyantara vritti; and staṁbha vritti.

Bāhya vṛtti is external activity. This means the activity of breathing out i.e. exhalation. Ābhyantara vṛtti is internal activity, bringing the air into you i.e. inhalation. Staṁbha vṛtti is stationary activity, no movement. This is breath holding. You stop the breath. You make the breath stationary.

These are the three breath activities: external, internal, stationary. Prānāyāma consists of deliberate control over exhalation, inhalation, and breath holding.

(Normally in prāṇāyāma breath holding refers to antah kumbhaka or holding after inhale. Later Hatha Yogis introduced holding after exhale. See discussion under The Fourth Prāṇāyāma.)

Deśa

What about your attention? Where do you control the breath? Deśa means a place or a spot. So deśa refers to the place in your body where you control the breath. You can control the breath in the throat (ujjayi); you can control the breath in the nostril (nadi shodana); you can control the breath at the tip of the tongue (śitalī).

When you hold the breath where should you have your attention? After inhalation when you hold the breath where do you feel it? You feel the breath in the chest. Your attention is in the heart when you do antah kumbhaka. When you start your exhalation you start feeling the movement from the lower abdomen. The diaphragm moves, the abdomen moves, the pelvic floor moves, the rectal muscles also come into play. When you exhale and hold the breath out and do mula and uddiyana bandha the attention will have to go to the rectal region and the navel region. So your attention has to change to different places. Your attention will vary depending on which aspect of prāṇāyāma you practice. Deśa refers to all these things.

Kāla

Kāla means time, duration. When you do prānāyāma the next parameter to look for is kāla. Prāṇāyāma is always done with a time measure in it. How long am I going to inhale? How long am I going to hold the breath? How long am I going to exhale? How long am I going to hold the breath out? All these come under the parameter kāla.

There are different types of prānāyāma. When you have equal amounts of inhalation and exhalation it is called samavṛitti prāṇāyāma. When you have a different inhalation/exhalation ratio then it is known as viṣamavṛitti prāṇāyāma. There are different types of prāṇāyāma depending on the kāla or time duration for the different aspects of your breathing.

If it is samavṛitti prāṇāyāma it will be equal inhalation and exhalation. If it is viṣamavṛitti prāṇāyāma the inhalation/exhalation ratios will vary. Suppose you inhale for some time, hold the breath four times as long, and exhale twice as long as the inhale, this is a viṣamavṛitti ratio 1:4:2. But if you inhale for five seconds, hold the breath for five seconds, exhale for five seconds, it is called samavṛitti prāṇāyāma.

Saṅkhya

Saṅkhya means count, number of times. How many times do I do prāṇāyāma during one sitting? Three prāṇāyāmas, ten prāṇāyāmas? It can be up to 80 prāṇāyāmas according to certain authors. Patañjali doesn't want to go into those details. He asks us to refer to other texts.

Sankalpa

Saṅkhya means the number of times you have to do prāṇāyāma in one sitting. You decide this in advance. You don't just sit down and do as many as you feel like. One has to start the Yoga practice with a sankalpa: I am going to do prāṇāyāma for so many times...Once you've made up your mind you cannot change. This is what Patañjali means by saṁkhya.

And, of course, the same holds true for deśa and kala.

(You may need a week and/or a teacher to try various prāṇāyāmas, ratios, etc. to find the one that is comfortable for you. But then, once you've settled down, you should not change during the practice. You should not allow the mind to play around.)

Total Attention

One reason why prāṇāyāma is very important is it forces your mind to be totally with the practice. Drsṭa is attention; paridrsṭo is total attention. You have to practice prāṇāyāma with total attention. Your attention should be completely in all these factors.

When you do prāṇāyāma what happens? the mind gets involved in the breathing activity. The mind should be totally with the practice. You can't be thinking of something else and practicing prāṇāyāma. Have you tried to do prāṇāyāma while thinking of something else? It's very difficult.

(That is why in VK we try to use the breathing so that the mind also will be with the breath. Mind will be with the breath, breath will be with your movement so that the mind and the body will be in union, in unison. That is what is mentioned in the YS in the sutras connected with the āsanas.)

Dirgha

Dirgha means long. I can inhale the breath for one second, hold the breath for one second, exhale for two seconds. That is not prāṇāyāma. Patañjali says you make it dirgha, very long.

Normally, when you practice prāṇāyāma over a period of time you should be able to do prāṇāyāma at the rate of two breaths per minute. This would be very good. But if it is three or even four breaths per minute it is ok. There are yogis who are able to do just one breath per minute. If they want to practice 18 prāṇāyāmas they will take about 18 minutes to do it. For most people who practice prāṇāyāma regularly it is possible to do 80 breaths in one hour's time. You develop an enormous amount of patience if you practice prāṇāyāma.

Sukṣma

Prāṇāyāma should not be heavy breathing. It should be sukṣma, subtle. Nice, smooth, long inhalation and exhalation.

Long and Smooth

The breathing should be long and smooth. You find instructions in other books such as the Upanishads. When you inhale the breath should be like drinking water through a straw or the stem of a blue water lily. Exhalation should be like pouring oil, a continuous stream. Patañjali indicates these by dīrgha and sūkṣma. This is the quality of the breath.

Breath Holding Necessary

So, for prāṇāyāma the various factors that have to be considered are contained in this sutra: any prāṇāyāma should include long, controlled inhalation; long, controlled breath holding; long, controlled exhalation. All three must be there, only then can it be called prāṇāyāma. If I merely inhale and exhale, even long inhalation, exhalation, it is not considered to be prāṇāyāma. It becomes prāṇāyāma when you do long inhalation, exhalation with breath holding.

Different Types of Prāṇāyāma

Different yogis have come out with different prāṇāyāmas. According to Śaṇkara the number of prāṇāyāmas is countless. There are so many yogis; they have come out with so many different types of prāṇāyāma. It is not really possible to count the number of prāṇāyāma techniques available according to Śaṅkara.

Every time you do prāṇāyāma you have to decide whether you want to do ujjayi prāṇāyāma or nadi shodana prāṇāyāma or anuloma or pratiloma, whatever. There are different types of prāṇāyāma. Most of the better known types of prāṇāyāma are viṣamavṛitti prāṇāyāma. Different sages have come out with different ratios for prāṇāyāma and they've all been accepted and are found in several of the older texts.

Here Patañjali says prāṇāyāma varies depending on where you control the breath, how long you control the breath, and also how many times you do prāṇāyāma.

The Self and the Prāṇa are Friends

According to Krishnamacharya the Self and the prāṇa are friends. The prāṇasthāna and the jivasthāna are said to be very close. So, if you are able to locate the prāṇasthāna and practice prāṇāyāma it produces a great relaxation to the mind. You feel extremely relaxed once you start doing prāṇāyāma.

The Fourth Prāṇāyāma

There are four activities in prāṇāyāma. One is rechaka which is exhalation. The next is inhalation which is called puraka. Then after inhalation is over, when you hold the breath, it is called kumbhaka or antah kumbhaka. This is what Patañjali has explained earlier. Bāhya vritti is known as rechaka. Ābhyantara vritti is known as puraka. And then staṁbha vṛtti is known as antah kumbhaka, when you hold the breath after inhale. These three parameters Patañjali has already discussed. This is the normal prāṇāyāma most people do.

Now, in sutra II.51, Patañjali talks about another parameter of prāṇāyāma which is something special. It is called the 4th type of prāṇāyāma or caturthaḥ.

Caturthaḥ means the fourth. Inhalation, exhalation, and breath holding are the first three breath activities.

The most common interpretation of this sutra is: in the fourth state there is no exhalation and no inhalation. Bāhya means external. What is external activity? It is exhalation. Ābhyantara is the internal activity, inhalation. Viṣaya means object. Here it refers to air, the breathing. Ākṣepī means removed from contention. If you can stop the breath without regard to inhalation or exhalation, that is if you can stop the breath at random, it is called kevala kumbhaka. It is stopping the breath without any consideration of inhalation or exhalation, just stopping the breath at any point. That is, you've got to stop the breath at will. This is called kevala kumbhaka.

Now Patañjali says if you can hold the breath, without inhalation or exhalation, it is a 4th kind of prāṇāyāma. The fourth one is random breath holding. Many people and texts consider kevala kumbhaka to be the fourth kind of prāṇāyāma. This is one school of thought. This is the first interpretation: kevala kumbhaka.

Kevala means alone. That particular kumbhaka is not associated with either inhalation or exhalation. Kevala kumbhaka is breath holding which is not preceded or followed by a specific aspect of breathing like inhalation or exhalation.

There are yogis who suddenly stop their inhalation or their exhalation. They suddenly stop their breath. It is neither preceded by an inhalation, which would be called antah kumbhaka, nor is it preceded by an exhalation, which would be called bāhya kumbhaka. At any time, the yogi decides ok I want to hold the breath. In fact, in the olden days when the yogi decided it was time to go he would hold the breath and leave the body.

The second interpretation:

There is a different interpretation for this sutra, a second understanding for what constitutes the fourth kind of prāṇāyāma.

In the prāṇāyāma that we normally practice we don't hold the breath out. In conventional prāṇāyāma, when you want to do prāṇāyāma before Gayatri japa and all that, you inhale, hold the breath, exhale, and then start your inhalation. Normally breath holding after exhale is not the conventional type of prāṇāyāma. But Haṭha yogis have introduced the bāhya kumbhaka or the breath holding after exhalation. According to some schools this sutra refers to bāhya kumbhaka. This is the second interpretation. Bāhya vṛtti is exhalation, ābhyantara vṛtti is inhalation. If you can hold the breath between these two it is the fourth one, the caturtha. That is, you exhale completely, you have not started your inhalation, during that particular period of time when you hold the breath it is called the 4th prāṇāyāma which is known as bāhya kumbhaka.

Some schools refer to the 4th as kevala kumbhaka; other schools say it refers to bahya kumbhaka.

Sahita kumbhaka; kevala kumbhaka

Sahita kumbhaka is a khumbhaka where you have the inhalation and exhalation associated with it. Kevala kumbhaka is a breath holding which is not associated with inhalation and exhalation.

Summary

These are the sutras referring to the practice of prāṇāyāma: YS II.49, 50, and 51. The 49th sutra talks about the mechanics of prāṇāyāma. The 50th sutra gives you all the parameters associated with prāṇāyāma. The

51st sutra talks about another special prāṇāyāma. And, with this Patañjali stops the subject of the practice of prāṇāyāma.

Samantraka Prāṇāyāma

At this point I'd also like to mention there is another kind of prāṇāyāma which according to my guru and several of the texts is very important. That prāṇāyāma is known as samantraka prāṇāyāma. That is, a prāṇāyāma done with mantra. This is a very popular prāṇāyāma. Several of the texts say samantraka prāṇāyāma is one thousand times more beneficial for the mind than amantraka prāṇāyāma.

Amantraka prāṇāyāma is the prāṇāyāma you normally do in a Haṭha Yoga class, if you do prāṇāyāma at all. You inhale, hold the breath, exhale. However there are some schools where they teach how to do prāṇāyāma with a mantra. Most likely you chant the mantra when you hold the breath in. But there are some schools where they chant the mantra after they exhale. And, there are some schools where they chant the mantra as you inhale and as you exhale. Different schools talk about using mantra in different ways.

According to Manu Smṛti there is a prāṇāyāma mantra which should be chanted when you hold the breath. When you hold the breath after inhalation you chant the mantra which consists of three parts: the vyahritis, the gayatri mantra, and a final portion called siras where you keep your consciousness with the sahasrāra and chant the last portion of the mantra. (You can hear this mantra chanted on Ramaswami's website: vinyasakrama.com.) With this the prāṇāyāma mantra is complete. It has a beautiful meaning. And if you can be in tune with that mantra it becomes a complete experience.

Then there are other mantras. If you are a Saivite, a Siva worshiper, you use a Siva mantra. They used the mantra, "Siva, Siva". They say that a certain amount of time and then this becomes the prāṇāyāma mantra for Saivites. Likewise there are other mantras which are used.

By yamaniyama you have normalized your relationship with the external world, then with āsana you are able to sit in a posture for a long period of time, with prāṇāyāma the mind becomes satvic, and then, during the prāṇāyāma you chant a mantra. Then that is known as samantraka prāṇāyāma.

Benefits

If you practice prāṇāyāma what are the benefits?

YS II.52 says that the practice of prāṇāyāma reduces the veil or covering of the light or clarity of the mind which is sattva. The veil that prevents you from seeing properly is reduced. It goes down gradually and eventually it is not there, meaning its affect is not there.

Āvaraṇa means a veil. It means surrounding or blocking the view. If you blindfold me it's called āvaraṇa. Āvaraṇa is a term used in other texts to refer to tamas; prakāśa refers to sattva. It is the āvarana which covers the prakāśa or light which is removed by prāṇāyāma. The use of prāṇāyāma helps to reduce the tamo guna.

The satvic aspect of the mind is completely blocked by the tamasic aspect of the mind. Āvarana is the tamo guna. The benefit arising out of prāṇāyāma is that the darkness of the mind which is called āvaraṇa is reduced or destroyed.

So for your mind to become satvic by the reduction of tamas, Patañjali says practice prāṇāyāma.

Earlier Patañjali said that the benefit from āsana practice is you will not be affected so easily by the pairs of opposites like heat and cold. The intolerance of the pairs of opposites is said to be rajas. That is, we have seen previously that the practice of āsana reduces the dvandva which refers to rajas. Āsana practice reduces the rajo guna. Here Patañjali says prāṇāyāma reduces the tamas aspect of the mind.

So the practice of āsana and prāṇāyāma reduce the rajo and tamo gunas and the space now becomes taken up by sattva. Once the system is rid of rajas and tamas the whole system becomes satvic and then such a mind is fit for the antaranga sadhanas, the internal practices Patañjali is going to talk about.

The next benefit is dhāraṇā, the first step of meditation, the first step of internal practice. By prāṇāyāma the mind is made fit for dhāraṇā. Only a sattvic mind is able to do dhāranā. The fitness of the mind for meditation is also ensured by prāṇāyāma practice.

In YS II.53, yogyatā means fitness, one who is fit. By the practice of prāṇāyāma the mind or chitta becomes fit for dhāranā. Dhāranā comes from the root dhṛ to support. So does dharma, some order which can support a particular system. So, II.53 says the mind becomes fit to contain something. If the tamas is there it doesn't allow any idea to come in. When rajas is there because the mind is fickle it is unable to hold on to anything. If both rajas and tamas have been removed (through asana and prāṇāyāma) the mind is able to hold onto any object, any subtle object, any subtle idea.

So, what do you get by prāṇāyāma practice? The tamo guna comes down, your mind becomes clearer and clearer, and not only that, the mind becomes fit for meditation.

Practice Āsana and Prāṇāyāma Together

For these reasons, Krishnamacharya used to keep saying: regularly practice āsana and prāṇāyāma together. Don't just practice āsana and go away. You practice āsanas, rajas has come down; practice prāṇāyāma, tamas has come down; then make use of your mind for meditation.

Patañjali says you need a proper āsana before you can do prāṇāyāma. So, āsana will have to be mastered. You have to find a seated posture where you can sit for a long period of time. All the effort you put in for āsana practice is to ultimately make you able to sit and be steady and comfortable for a long period of time.

Supposing I want to do a half hour or a one hour prāṇāyāma practice, for that one hour of time I don't want to be shifting from one side to the other, I want to remain steady and without discomfort. Steady does not mean I have to endure pain. The posture should be such that I'll be able to remain there for a long period of time without any discomfort.

From this you can see that if you practice āsana and prāṇāyāma together both rajas and tamas will have come down and your mind is fit for meditation, fit for dhāranā.

Breath in Āsana is not Prāṇāyāma

We don't do prāṇāyāma during āsana practice. Prāṇāyāma involves breath holding. In our āsana practice we make use of the breath: we focus the attention on the breath. And, the breath is synchronized with the movement so that the mind is going to be with the whole exercise. What we do in āsana practice, in Vinyasa Krama, is only rechaka and puraka, inhalation and exhalation, synchronized inhalation and exhalation. Only when you introduce the element of breath holding does it become prāṇāyāma. Patañjali says gati vicchedaḥ prāṇāyāmaḥ. When we hold the breath for a moment or two in āsana that is not prāṇāyāma for prāṇāyāma breath holding can sometimes run to about 20 or 25 seconds when you chant with a mantra. We don't hold the breath that long in āsana. So normally in Vinyasa Krama the breathing we do is not called prāṇāyāma

Prep for Meditation

If you want to be successful with your meditation you must first practice āsana and prāṇāyāma. If you practice āsana and prāṇāyāma don't waste the effort, sit down and meditate because you have already prepared yourself in such a way that your mind is satvic. Make use of the satvic mind and develop the capacity for ekāgra, one pointedness.

If you try to meditate without āsana and prāṇāyāma practice your mind will continue to be in either a rajasic or tamasic mold or a combination of these two and that is not a conducive state for mediation. Without the reduction of rajas and tamas you cannot meditate. If the rajas and tamas come down then you are fit for meditaion. Just as we make the body fit we must make the mind fit.

There are a few who are born yogis. They can meditate at the drop of a hat. But, for most of us when we close our eyes all the thoughts come back. We watch all those thoughts. So when you meditate you continue to have the same kind of experience you normally have. The mind has not been prepared for meditation. Anyone who wants to meditate without the preparation will not succeed.

An Integrated Approach

There is no point in your doing the higher yoga practice without preparing yourself with the preliminary yoga practices. On the other hand, if you do all the preliminary things, make use of it so that you can go to the higher practice of yoga. Unfortunately we don't find that.

There's a group which meditates without all these preparations; there's another group which practices āsana and they don't go further. But in ashtanga yoga it is an integrated approach. You have all the aṅgas that are necessary. You can start anywhere. If you are already practicing yamaniyama then you can start your āsana prāṇāyāma practice. If you are not doing any of those things before you start your āsana practice, practice yama niyama to some extent. Once you have imbibed these ideas of yama niyama your āsana practice will be successful, your prāṇāyāma practice will be successful and then you can go for meditation.

Waste Not, Want Not

Even though the mind has become sattvic, because the mind has been getting a lot of pleasure from the indriyas, things that we see, things that we hear, etc., once you complete your practice and you open your eyes and return to the everyday world, the mind gets led out through the senses and you become distracted. And all your efforts, all that you have done to reduce tamas and rajas, are slowly reduced and all the benefits you have gained will be lost in the next half an hour. So, to take advantage of what you have gained through asana and pranayama Patañjali suggests: why don't you go ahead and practice dhāranā.

There are people who spend a lot of their time in āsana and prāṇāyāma practice and people who practice āsana and then don't do prāṇāyāma. They prepare themselves and then don't make use of it. When you prepare yourself through the practice of āsana and prāṇāyāma you've got to use it, follow it up with some kind of a meditation practice.

10

Pratyāhāra

Definition

The next aṅga, called pratyāhāra, is not a great one, but, at the same time, it is a very useful aṅga. Pratyāhāra is the name of the fifth aṅga of aṣṭaṅga yoga. What does it mean? Patañjali defines it as: the senses not used or not connected with their own objects. It means the eyes do not see, the ears do not hear, etc. You try to seal all the senses.

Prati means against; prati means stopping it. Āhāra means to take something (in).

Āhāra

Normally, the word āhāra is used for food. If I don't take food it is called pratyāhāra. But here the word āhāra is much more comprehensive. It refers to all the "food" I take for my various senses. It refers to everything that we take in from the outside world. What we eat, what we see, what we hear, what we touch. Don't let all the senses to go after their objects as they normally do. This practice, over a period of time, leads to the senses being controlled by the mind.

What is the food for my ears? I hear a lot of things. What is the food for my eyes? I see a lot of things. Likewise all the senses take a lot of things from the outside world. The outside world provides a lot of information, a lot of stimulus, to these senses. Normally, our senses are always active. When somebody calls we immediately hear them. But, if for a period of time you say ok, I don't want to hear anything, I don't want to see anything. Shut everything out. I won't hear anything; I won't see anything. That period of time when you shut out all the indriyas is called pratyāhāra.

Senses Are Controlled

Why do you want to do it? Patañjali's going to tell you why it is necessary. Because having done āsana and prāṅāyāma, your mind is satvic. Now what do you do? To take advantage of what you have gained through āsana and prāṇāyāma Patañjali suggests you go ahead and practice dhāranā. Only these holes, these senses start dragging the mind away from dhāranā. Before you even start thinking of dhāranā, as soon as you complete your āsana and prāṅāyāma practice what do you do? You immediately turn to your neighbor and your neighbor turns to you and you start talking about oh, where shall we go, what shall we do? The senses have already started dragging us. To help with this Patañjali introduces pratyāhāra (II.54), to make the senses turn inward.

For one hour you have been alone, practicing alone. The moment you stop the senses start dragging you. But for a period of time we don't want the senses to drag us. So the yogis have devised methods called pratyāhāra. Ok, for a short period of time I am not going to engage the senses in their respective activities. If you can find out a particular procedure by which you can achieve this that particular procedure is called pratyāhāra.

I don't want objects to again drag the senses because my mind also will be dragged through the senses. I worked hard for an hour or so. I've done my āsanas to reduce my rajas. I've done another ten, fifteen minutes of prāṅāyāma to reduce my tamas. I don't want the senses to play spoil sport. I don't want that to happen. So, I need a simple procedure by which I can arrest the senses and stop them from dragging me away.

I won't use my ears to hear anything. I won't use my eyes to see anything. When you stop these senses from acting, within a short period of time you feel as though there are no senses. They all merge with the mind which is a coordinating sense. All of them become part of the mind itself, at least for a short duration of time.

By the practice of pratyāhāra(II.55), all the indriyas become totally controlled.

Five Methods

There are different methods of pratyāhāra suggested such as lying down in shavasana and drawing your mind inward. In fact, there are five different pratyāhāra practices mentioned in the śāstras. In the system of Vinyasa Krama, Krishnamacharya suggested the method of shanmukhi mudra where you close your ears, eyes, etc., and then try to focus your attention on something inside, maybe the breath or some part of the body like the ajna chakra or the throat. The senses are not allowed to wander. We do this immediately after prāṇāyāma. It prepares you for dhāranā. According to Krishnamacharya, shanmuki mudra is perhaps the most affective method of pratyāhāra.

Normally, we train the body, we train the mind, but we don't interfere with the senses. Now Patañjali wants to do that. Make the senses not go after an object for a short period of time. That kind of training will have to be given. Of course, it is really the mind which will have to be trained. Shanmukhi mudra has been given in several of the old Upanishads for this.

The five types of Pratyāhāra:

1. Effort of drawing the senses from their respective sense objects (Shanmukhi mudra).
2. Seeing everything as an extension of the (Supreme) Soul – (Vedantic approach).
3. Surrendering the results of doing one's duties to

the Lord -- (Karma Yoga).

4. Avoiding engagement of the senses with their respective objects as a matter of habit (abstinence)

5. Focusing on the 18 vital spots (marmasthana) in the body sequentially (from crown to toe and toe to crown) usually in Shavasana.

Benefit

What is the benefit of the practice of pratyāhāra? According to Yoga, out of this practice of pratyāhāra all the senses are controlled by the mind.

There are eleven indriyas: the five karma indriyas, the five jñāna indriyas and the mind. Over time, through the practice of pratyāhāra the mind becomes not easily distracted by the senses. The senses by themselves do not have any motive. They just allow the input, the various āhāra, to go in.

The mind is the superior sense, the eleventh sense, which controls both the karma indriyas and the jñānendriyas. The karma indriyas being the arms, the legs, etc. and the jñānendriyas are the eyes, the ears, etc. The sense organs and the organs or action come under the control of the mind. This is not normally the case for over a period of time we have allowed the reverse to happen. We have allowed these senses to control the mind.

When we are sitting down in a room and somebody talks there are some people who will be so nicely concentrating they won't even hear. But most of us will hear. This is because the mind is easily distracted.

So, if you practice pratyahara regularly over a period of time the senses will come under the control of the mind rather than the senses distracting the mind. This is the benefit of pratyāhāra practice.

If you practice like this after some time you feel as if there are no senses. The senses merge with the mind which is the controller of all the senses. After pratyāhāra, if we keep the eyes closed, it is not as though the objects aren't there, but even if there's a smell or a sound, etc. it's as though they don't exist.

On Your Own

Once you start your pratyāhāra (and then proceed to meditation) you are on your own. Not even your guru comes and tells you what to do. Once you start your meditation everybody will have to keep quiet including your own guru. He's outside this practice.

You practice meditation for five, ten minutes. Then go back to your teacher: this is what happened, what should I do? But you do not receive instructions during the time you are meditating. The moment some other sounds or some instructions start coming, as happens in guided meditation, then it's a different practice.

Baharanga Sadhana Complete

So, we've had prāṇāyāma to bring the breath under control, asana to bring the body under control, now we have pratyāhāra to bring the senses under control.

This completes the baharanga sadhana.

11

Antaraṅga Sādhana

(meditation)

Meditation According to the Yoga Sutra

According to the YS, what you meditate on is not the main thing. You must be able to bring your mind to an object and then go into Samādhi on that particular object. That is what is important, that you develop that capability because it is not sufficient to meditate on one object. After all, there are 24 tattvas. We should be able to go into Samadhi on one particular object, master it, know everything about it, and then you go to the next subtler one.

Two Ways To Look At It

There are two ways to look at it. If you are meditating on your favorite deity then the object becomes very important. You are going to focus your attention on the object and there is nothing else to think about. So that object is the ultimate goal. But here, in the YS, Patañjali talks about starting with any simple object. You meditate upon that. Once you are able to develop the capacity to be focused on that without being distracted by anything else then you have developed the ekāgra capacity. You keep on using it to understand higher and higher principles.

Antaraṅga Sādhana

The third chapter of the YS is on Antaraṅga Sādhana, practices which are internal. Antaraṅga means internal; Sādhana means practice or effort. From here on it is an exercise for the mind alone. It is not a physical exercise; it is not a breathing exercise; it is not controlling the senses. No, now you are going to work with the mind.

Now the yogi has come to a stage where through the practice of asana and prāṇāyāma he has been able to greatly reduce rajas and tamas. By reducing rajas and tamas he has been able to make sattva the predominant quality. A sattvic mind is necessary for the antaraṅga sadhana. To be able to gain nirodha requires a sattvic mind (achieved by the practice of aṣṭāṅga yoga). Chapter III is for those who have rajas and tamas under great control. If you try and practice antaraṅga sadhana without reducing rajas and tamas you are not likely to succeed.

You have already prepared the mind very well. Āsana, Prāṅāyāma, yama, niyama, control of the diet, all these things have helped to make your mind satvic. Now you have a very fit, yogic mind with which you can work.

Progress

The progress that you make in antaraṅga sadhana is by and large the responsibility of the individual. Up to pratyāhāra a lot can be taught by the teacher. But from here on it is the responsibility of the student to apply the techniques for progress. The teacher can tell you how to go about it according to Patañjali, but the effort must be made by the student.

Whether you make progress or not you know better than the teacher. You are the only person who knows what is happening in your mind. You are the only person who can manipulate your mind, who can modify your mind. That's why they call it Antaraṅga Sādhana. In the olden days antaraṅga meant something secret. Nobody knows what happens in your mind.

The First Stage

Patañjali does not simply say go and mediate. Instead he divides the antaraṅga sadhana into three stages. The first stage is called dhāraṇā. Dhāraṇā is the starting point of your meditation practice.

Patañjali uses the word dhāraṇā as a technical term. Dhāraṇā means to support something, to remain steadfast. It comes from the root dhṛ, to support. If the mind is able to support an idea, if the mind is able to stick to an idea for a considerable length of time, if the mind does not deviate from that object or place, then that particular exercise of the mind is called dhāraṇā.

Normally, when the mind is rajasic it jumps from one object to another. That is the manifestation of rajo guna. But Vyasa in his commentary says that we all have the capacity for dhāraṇā.

This is the first step of the internal practice, a practice that is taking place inside you, inside your mind.

The Sixth Aṇga

The sixth aṅga of Yoga, the sixth aspect of Yoga, is known as dhāraṇā.

Dhāraṇā

The binding of the mind at (to) a place is called dhāraṇā (III.1).

Patañjali uses the word "place". He could have used the word "object" but, there are places which are not objects e.g. a spot in the body. It could as well be a mantra. Sound can be regarded as an object or place. So, the "object" of meditation can be a spot in the body, a chakra, an object outside the body, the sun, the moon, an icon or idol of a deity, sound of a mantra, light, breath, etc. It should be something elevating. (Mantra may be easier because you can go on repeating it. Even so the mind may wander.)

Now for people who follow chakra meditation this place that is talked about could be the mūlādhāra chakra, the svādhisthāna chakra, the maṇipūra chakra, anāhata, vishuddhi, ājña, or sahasrāra depending upon where you can tie your mind.

On the other hand, Vyasa says you can focus your attention on an external object. If you are used to icon worship, you have the icon. It can be a beautiful, divine object. It may be a flame. Patañjali gives you a number of choices. He doesn't say to focus your attention on this or that, focus on an object or a sound. It can be any of those things. Patañjali does not say this is a good meditation or that one is better. This is up to you and your guru. Patañjali doesn't want to interfere with that. He only says repeated attempts to tie the mind to an object or a place is called dhāraṇā.

Patañjali gives a large number of alternatives. In Vyasa's commentary he says that any object can be taken. The only qualification is that the object you choose should be uplifting. It may be Om, one of the chakras, a light in your heart or between the eyebrows. There are so many methods suggested.

Look at the object. See to it that you bring your mind to the same object repeatedly. That is the capability of the mind that I don't have now. But the mind has got it. It's a dormant capability. I want to bring it up.

Binding the Mind

What is meant by binding? You start focusing your attention at a place. Because the natural tendency of the mind is to deviate, it wanders. So, you bring the mind back to that same place again. Again it wanders. Again bring it back. This is binding. It is like tying a calf to a pole. You bring it back to the same spot over and over again. When that is done, after a while, the mind will start staying with the object for a longer period of time. This we can observe and evaluate.

So dhāraṇā refers to repeated attempts by the yogi to focus his/her attention on an object. Once you start meditating like this, if you have excessive rajas or tamas the mind will never settle down. But now the Yogi is in a position to succeed because he has reduced his rajas and tamas.

The mind is not bound to a place now. It goes from one place to another, one thought to another, one object to another, absolutely uncontrolled. Now, I'm binding it. I am tying it to an object. My mind is there. I close my eyes and then I start thinking of an object. My mind goes away. Then, what do I do? I bring my mind back, try to tie it to the object. Again it goes away. Again I bring it back. This effort is called dhāraṇā.

Keep It Simple

It is best to begin with a simple object, as simple as possible because we are trying to develop a skill. The goal is to develop the skill of concentration. Once the skill is developed we can use this skill to meditate on, for instance, the 24 tattvas.

Even with a very simple object the mind naturally has a tendency to jump from the object to thoughts about that object. We want to reduce this jumping back and forth until we reach a point where the mind is with the object alone. We want the mind to settle on the object or place or sound.

So it is not advisable, in the beginning, to choose a concept such as heaven or infinity as the object for our meditation. These concepts are vague and the mind will jump from thought to thought about them. It is best to start with a simpler object to gain the skill of concentration. Once we have this skill more complex concepts can be tackled such as the kośas as the Vedantins do, meditating on each kośa in turn, realizing that it is not the Self.

Bringing the Mind Under Control

Dhāranā consists of repeated attempts to bring your mind to an object. Normally we don't do it. Normally we allow the mind to take its own course. True sometimes, because it is a requirement, you focus your mind for a short period of time but then it wanders. You don't bring the mind under voluntary control at all. Having brought the body under control by āsana, having brought the breath under control by prāṇāyāma, having brought the indriyas under control by pratyāhāra, Patañjali now wants you to bring the mind under control by the practice of antaraṅga sādhana.

The first way to control the mind is to bring the mind to the same object over and over and over again. Now you are controlling the mind. How do I know if I can control the mind? If I can keep the mind attached to the same object for a considerable amount of time that means I have been able to control the mind.

In practical terms, suppose you want to meditate, you sit down, you close your eyes. One of the methods by which you can focus your attention is to take a mantra. Mantras are easy to use because you can go on repeating one. Mantra also is an object. It's a sound which the mind can be attached to. You keep on chanting the mantra over and over again.

You've got to choose a mantra that is useful to you. You should really like the mantra. There's no point taking a mantra whose meaning you don't know or if you don't know whether it is good for you or not.

So you start the chanting of the mantra. You chant the mantra for a short period of time. Then what happens? Without your knowledge the mind will wander. Sometimes, even with a mantra, the mind wanders. Why does the mind wander? Because that's what it is used to. Then what do you do? You realize the mind has wandered and you come back to the mantra. You bring the mind back. That's the only effort you have to make. I'm not going to fight with my mind. I'm going to watch my mind. The moment the mind wanders I want to bring it back.

Like a Baby Sitter

Supposing you are a baby sitter, you don't have to keep the baby in your lap all the time. You just have to be watchful. You have to see that the baby does not go out of the room. Similarly, we don't want the mind to go out of the object. If it goes away bring it back. Tie it around. Again it goes away, bring it back. Through this repeated effort over time then, like the child, the mind also will settle down to the same object.

Japa Mala

Patañjali doesn't talk about japa here. But japa can be a beginning if you want to use a mala. For some people using a japa mala could be helpful. That is, you close your eyes and you keep on repeating your mantra. After you use the japa mala for some time you should be able to set it aside and meditate without it. But most people get stuck to the japa mala all their lives. So, that is a risk.

If it is a religious practice then you are not going to think of any other mantra. All your life you are going to be practicing with only that particular mantra. Ok, then that is the end of the whole story. But if you want to develop the capacity for meditation, you take a mantra, keep on repeating the mantra until you are able to get into some kind of dhyāna with that particular mantra.

In dhyāna it is not a repetition. There what you try to do is bring you mind to the same object over and over. Patañjali doesn't talk about number of times. He doesn't say how many times you have to do it. But, that could be helpful. Using a japa mala could be helpful for some people.

Mantra Japa and Mantra Dhyāna

There are two things: mantra japa and mantra dhyāna. Mantra japa is repetition. You keep on repeating the mantra. In mantra dhyāna you try to bring your mind to the object repeatedly. Watch for a period of time, if the mind wanders bring it back. This is the procedure Patañjali is talking about.

The yogi wants to transcend the mind. Ultimately he should be able to give up the mantra. The mantra is used so that the mind gets the capability of being absorbed in something without any distraction whatsoever.

Evaluating the Process

At the end of your dhāranā practice you look back and ask how many times did my mind wander? What was the duration of those detours? This will tell you the quality of your meditation. It also helps you know which thoughts are bothering you. Those thoughts that come and interfere are the ones that are uppermost in your mind. Over a period of time you try and solve those problems.

If you keep on doing this, one day you will find that over the entire duration of dhāraṇā the mind is with the object. When that happens we go to the next stage: dhyāna.

So, in dhāranā you've got to increase the span of concentration. You can't force it on your mind. What you have to observe is: am I increasing the span of concentration? Is the number of distractions coming down? And, is the duration of the distractions coming down?

Two Reasons for Difficulty

There are two reasons why dhāranā may be difficult. One is the presence of rajas and tamas, especially rajas. For this we may do more āsana, eat less rajasic food, etc. The other reason is: my mind has never done this. And, because it has never done this my mind goes back to its old habit of running away. So, what do you do? You develop this samskara. You develop this particular practice. You keep working on it. Your mind will slowly learn to be with the object.

It does not depend on how intelligent I am. It is a particular capability of the mind which I don't have, just like learning how to ride a bicycle or a horse. I need some time. I may be a nobel laureate but, I don't know how to pedal a cycle. I have to learn that.

We should not think we cannot get it. Every mind is capable of this. That's what Vyasa says in his commentary to YS I.1: Sārva bhauma chittasya dharma.

Dhyāna

Literally, dhyāna means to constantly think of something. (Always on a higher or uplifting object.)

Patañjali explains dhyāna in YS III.2: If the the chitta vritti (or the tendency of the mind or the focus of the mind or the flow of the mind) is with the object (or in the same place) continually for the duration of your practice then it is called dhyāna.

When you keep on practicing dhāranā over time it matures to this next stage called dhyāna. Slowly, over a period of time, because you have already created a proper condition for the mind to be practicing this dhāranā your mind will be with the object for a much longer time. Instead of running away after two or three seconds, it may perhaps stay with the object for one minute. Again it may go away. Previously, if the mind wandered it wandered for a long period of time. It used to take not a five minute break but, a half hour break. Now, after some time the break is less. After a very short period of time you realize that the mind has wandered and you are able to bring the mind back. So, the span of your distraction starts coming down. The frequency of your distraction also starts coming down. And then, over a period of time, you'll find that one day the mind is with the object for the entire duration of time you are meditating. And, that is called dhyāna. That is the second stage of meditation.

The next day it may not be so good because the rest of the time you spent distracting your mind or you ate some rajasic food which is not satvic, any number of reasons. The mind still has lots of the old samskaras. But, at least you know you've made progress. You continue with the same practice for some more time and you'll find the quality of your meditation starts improving. Instead of the mind wandering most of the time, the mind will be with the object for most of the time. That itself is an improvement. So you keep on practicing and after some time the mind will be in dhyāna continually. There may be the occasional distraction but, by and large, your mind has now developed a new capability.

If the mind is going to be with the same object continually, whether the object be gross or subtle, then it is called dhyāna. If the mind is going to be with the object continually, only one object, without interruption, without being distracted by any other object, that particular state is called dhyāna. If for the entire duration of meditation the mind flows through the same object continually then that state is called dhyāna.

In this case, while you are meditating on an object, you are aware, as an individual that you are mediating upon that.

Difference Between Dhāranā and Dhyāna

You see the difference between dhāranā and dhyāna? In dhāranā the mind goes away from the object, it doesn't yet have the capability of staying continually.

There is nothing mysterious about meditation so far as Patañjali is concerned. He has divided it into three stages so that we will be able to understand what is going on in the mind.

End Where You Start

Suppose you start focusing on an object and stay with it for some time and then the mind goes to another object which the mind likes and stays with that -- This happens when you have too many mantras – this is not dhyāna. You should end with the object you started with.

Necessity of the Previous Step

Dhyāna comes only by way of the previous step, dhāranā. In the previous step you make an enormous amount of effort to remain with the object. In dhāranā a lot of effort is required because the mind is not used to it. So we have to develop the particular samskara, the particular habit of the mind.

You make the effort. If you don't make the effort dhyāna will not come. Dhyāna, or remaining with the object, cannot take place without the earlier step of your making the effort, and keeping on making the effort, to be with the object. We never do that in our normal way of life. So, Patañjali is talking about a different kind of capability which the mind has but which we have not developed.

Samādhi

The next stage is samādhi. Patañjali explains it in sutra III.3: The same object and the object alone shines in the mind. It alone is seen in the mind. You even forget yourself. When the meditator sees only the object, when the mind is full with the object as if the meditator is not there then Patañjali calls it samādhi.

So in the next stage you are still with the same object and you are able to remain with the same object continuously for the period of time you are meditating and now what happens? That object alone shines or is seen in your mind as though you are not there seeing it.

You know normally when you are seeing something you are aware that you are seeing it. But here, after some time you forget even yourself, you forget that you are watching. Only the object remains in your mind. And that stage is called samādhi. It is the third stage of meditation.

Sometimes when we go to a concert we forget ourselves for a few moments. But that is only momentary. In Samadhi, the Yogi is able to forget himself for a considerable amount of time. And, he is able to get into Samadhi every time he meditates on the object.

Three Components of Experience

All our experiences have three components. One is the memory of the object, the second is the object itself, and the third is the name of the object.

(Holds up a bottle.) When I see this I know it is a bottle. How do I know that? I know it because it is already in my memory. The moment I see it I already have some memory of that. I am able to call it back.

The third component, the name, means as soon as you say the word "bottle" I am able to visualize the bottle.

So, there are three things: śabda, artha, jñanaṁ. Śabda means word, artha is object, and jñana is the memory of it.

Sometimes when you meditate all three get mixed up. Let's suppose I've got an object. I keep on seeing this object. And then suddenly I think it is a bottle. And then sometimes I even say, "bottle". Likewise when you use a mantra the same three components are also there.

If you are able to focus your attention on the same object even when all three, memory, object and name, are mixed up it is still samādhi. But it is an inferior samādhi. You should be able to separate all three.

Supposing I say, "bottle, bottle, bottle". I should be able to say the mantra "bottle" over a long period of time without thinking of a bottle. If I can do that it is a higher kind of meditation.

Three Stages of Meditation

So, there are three stages of mediation. In the first stage, there is a repeated attempt on the part of the meditator to focus attention on the object. In the second stage, the entire period of time the meditaion is taking place the meditator is with the object, there is no break (dhyāna). In the third stage the meditator forgets himself.

There is only one object. In the first stage I make a lot of effort to observe the object. In the second stage, I am able to remain with the object continuously for the duration of time I am meditating. In the third stage I even forget myself. The object is the same. I have not changed the object.

Saṁyama

If all three, dhāranā, dhyāna, samādhi are with respect to one object then Patañjali calls it saṁyama. All three should be on the same object.

Saṁ means complete; yama means control. There is a total control of the mind with the object. Saṁyama is the term used for meditation in the text.

If I get into samādhi on an object different from the one I started with then it is not saṁyama.

Sometimes what happens is: I am meditating on one object and then I'm able to go into Samādhi on that object. Next time, when I want to meditate on another object, I start with another object but, I wind up going back to the old Samādhi.

I've been able to meditate on this bottle. I'm able to go into Samādhi with this bottle. Next day I want to meditate on this iPod. I start meditating on this iPod and then by the time I complete my mediatation what is in my mind is the bottle. This is not saṁyama.

But, if my mind is going to start with the iPod and end with the iPod it is called saṁyama. If I start with the iPod and end with the bottle because I've meditated with the bottle before and gone into Samādhi with the bottle then it is not called saṁyama.

You must be able to stay with one particular object, get full knowledge of that object and only then move to another one. There are 24 principles. I meditate on one principle and realize this is not me. Then I go on to the next one. You start with gross objects, go to subtle objects.

This is a very important message of the YS. Your ability to go into samādhi should not bind you to that particular object. Why does Patañjali say this? Because many times what happens is you not only meditate on an object you get attached to that object.

The Capability

So try to get that capability. The capability is the important thing, not the object. We're trying to get the capability to focus our attention on different objects. So, start with a simple object, develop the capability to go into samādhi with that object. Know everything that is to be known about that object through your samādhi practice. This is called sāmprajñāta samādhi, a samādhi which helps us to completely understand an object. This is the samādhi we need to understand the true nature of one's own Self -- because it is so subtle.

The idea of Raja Yoga is to first develop the capability of going into samādhi on one object and then being able to transfer that capability to subtler and subtler objects.

12

Transformation

(Pariṇāma)

Three Different Pariṇāmas

Pariṇāma means transformation. Pariṇāma is not just a momentary thing. The mind is completely transformed.

Patañjali talks about three different pariṇāmas, three different transformations of the mind. They are: nirodha pariṇāma, samādhi pariṇāma, and ekāgratā pariṇāma.

As usual, Patañjali begins with the highest transformation, nirodha pariṇāma. Then he follows this with the second transformation, samādhi, and the third transformation, ekāgratā.

Vyutthāna

Once the yogi has developed the capability of saṁyama he is capable of extraordinary powers, called siddhis, such as levitation, walking on water, stopping the heart, and the rest, which normal people are not capable of. The siddhis all come about through the Yogi's mastery of concentration.

Vyutthāana means outgoing. Once the mind has the capability of acquiring various siddhis the mind develops a taste for them. The mind has a desire for the siddhis. This is what is meant here by vyutthāna.

Such a mind is called a vyutthita chitta. It is not trying to understand the nature of the Self but, because it already has the capability of going into samādhi that samādhi is used for supernatural powers. If the mind is going to be interested in this that particular mind is called vyutthita chitta, a mind which is after siddhis. Oh, I can walk on water. What do you do next? I can walk on fire.

These are all capabilities which you and I don't have that but a siddha does. Only the siddha uses that capability not to understand the nature of the Self and go into nirodha but to go after different kinds of siddhis. So, this is called vyutthita chitta, a mind which goes out. Our minds go out for worldly things.

So far as the siddha purusha is concerned his mind goes after extraordinary capabilities. He's not satisfied with becoming a city councilman; He wants to become the President. Likewise, here the mind goes after extraordinary capabilities but, not understanding the nature of the Self.

But these siddhis are not the ultimate goal of Yoga. The ultimate goal is nirodha. And, in fact, the siddhis become a distraction on the path to the ultimate goal. This is called vyutthāna.

Nirodha Pariṇāma

The first transformation Patañjali talks about is called nirodha pariṇama. Here the mind is transformed into a state of nirodha. Nirodha is the highest stage. This is the last transformation of the Yogi's mind. Patañjali mentions this first because this is the ultimate transformation, nirodha being the ultimate goal.

Two Saṁskāras Compared

In sutra III.9 Patañjali compares two saṁskāras, two states of mind, two kinds of people. One is the siddha, the person who goes after various siddhis, supernatural powers. Whereas there is another, a Yogi, whose mind is after understanding the nature of the Self. We are talking about the difference between the siddha purusha and the Yogi.

This mind has the capability, called saṃprajñāta samādhi, to understand all the various objects. Such a mind is able to understand the nature of the Self, and then a transformation can take place. And, that transformation is called nirodha pariṇāma.

This mind has two kinds of saṁskāras. The mind already has the capability to get into saṁyama, but still the mind has a taste for different siddhis, called vyutthāna. The other samskara is nirodha: No, I know what the nature of the Self is I do not want any of these siddhis.

What is the difference between these two? When my mind is a vyutthita chitta it goes after various siddhis. In the ultimate stage of nirodha none of the siddhis interest the mind any more because it has known the nature of the Self. Compared to that none of these siddhis are of any interest to the mind.

Once this takes place then the mind must slowly develop the saṁskāra, that is it should become habitual. One mind goes after siddhis habitually; another mind does not go after these siddhis habitually even though it has the capability. So, these two are compared.

For the first few days the mind says no, I am not interested in this. Then this tendency keeps on increasing. And, over a period of time the mind becomes full of this nirodha saṁskāra.

Abhibhava means subsiding. What subsides? The desire to know everything in the universe. That is vyutthita chitta. That goes on coming down. Over a period of time it comes down. The tendency to remain quiet within oneself starts and keeps on increasing. And then, ultimately, over a period of time, the mind is full of only the second set of saṁskāras.

Nirodha pariṇāma is described as vyutthāna going down and nirodha coming up moment after moment. The previous saṁskāras (siddhis) become weak (abhibhava) from not being used.

We want to reduce those saṁskāras which are outgoing, wanting to obtain siddhis. And the space is now taken up by nirodha. Slowly, the habit of going after siddhis is reduced and the tendency to remain in nirodha is increased. One comes down; the other goes up.

Then what happens? Every moment the mind is in a state of nirodha. This moment the mind is in a state of nirodha. After half an hour the mind is in a state of nirodha. Moment after moment after moment the mind remains in a state of nirodha. And when that takes place that is called pariṇāma, transformation.

A mind which has been going after various siddhis becomes a mind which is in the stage of nirodha. A siddha mind is transformed into a nirodha mind – a mind which is in nirodha. This is the ultimate transformation. This Patañjali calls the highest pariṇāma, the highest transformation. As is common in many texts, Patañjali states this first.

Every Mind has the Capability

Every chitta has the capability of going into nirodha just as in the previous stage every mind has the capability to go into saṁyama.

Absolute Peace

When that saṃskāra takes root, when the mind is totally transformed into nirodha, absolute peace flows (III.10). The mind of the Yogi is absolutely peaceful. It arises out of nirodha pariṇāma. It is not an experience.

In that state (nirodha) what does the Yogi feel? There is no experience. There is no bliss. There is no happiness. There is no sorrow. But, in such a mind, praśantavāhitā: absolute peace flows. That is, moment after moment there is absolute peace. Here peace has an entirely different meaning from satisfaction or happiness.

In that nirodha mind there is a continuous flow of absolute peace. As the mind remains in chitta vritti nirodha the mind remains in an absolute state of peace all the time. This moment my mind is in chitta vritti nirodha. My mind is in a state of peace. Next moment my mind is in chitta vritti nirodha, my mind is in a state of peace. There is a flow of peace, a flow of chitta vritti nirodha.

Once having known the nature of the Self, the mind is totally satisfied and has no further use for samādhi. The Yogi who was a siddha yogi has become a Raja Yogi.

Inside Job

Chitta vritti nirodha is not something which can be done from the outside. The mind has to go through the process of pariṇāma.

Cannot Reach Nirodha Pariṇāma Directly

But you cannot reach this stage directly. What is the previous stage?

Two Other Pariṇāmas

There are two other pariṇāmas referred to: Samādhi Pariṇāma and Ekāgratā Pariṇāma.

Samādhi Pariṇāma

We cannot go directly to nirodha. We must first have the samādhi saṃskāras we get from samādhi pariṇāma.

More accurate would have been saṃprajñāta samādhi pariṇāma or sabīja samādhi pariṇāma because here, in YS III.11, samādhi refers to the term saṃyama.

There are two different tendencies the mind has: going after many objects vs. going after one object. Sarvārthata is a mind which is after many objects due to rajas, i.e. a mind in a state of vikshipta. If instead the mind can be trained to focus on one object, come into samādhi on one object, and do so habitually, that kind of transformation is samādhi pariṇāma. The mind has this capability. It is not able to do this because of saṃskāras, old habits.

Patañjali wants the mind which is after many objects to deteriorate (kṣaya) and the mind focused on one object to arise (udayau). The previous tendency subsides: the other tendency comes up. The tendency to go after different objects comes down; keeping one object in your mind for the entire period of meditation comes up. When this takes place, when it becomes established as a saṃskāra, that transformation of the mind is called samādhi pariṇāma.

I've got to transform my mind from the tendency to go after many objects to the tendency to focus on one object and remain focused on that object for a long period of time until I'm able to obtain saṃyama on that object.

My mind which is slowly able to get into a stage of samādhi is transformed into a mind which can habitually go into a stage of samādhi. This transformation is the second transformation. It is a lower level of pariṇāma.

Ekāgratā Pariṇāma

Now Patañjali goes into the process of meditation itself. In the process of meditation in one moment, which we call the previous moment or the dying moment, my mind was with one object, and in the next moment my mind is with the same object. If the object is the same during the dying and uprising moment and I can do this habitually then that kind of pariṇāma is called ekāgratā pariṇāma.

Eka means one; agratā means in front of the mind. When you are able to keep one object in front of the mind habitually you have transformed the mind. Ekāgratā has become a saṃskāra. That is ekāgratā pariṇāma.

So, we look at our own thoughts. Every moment our thoughts change. I have one thought and in two or three moments another thought comes. This is how our mind functions. But, if the mind, which is thinking of different things at different moments, is able to remain with the same object moment after moment, and further if this becomes a habit, then that is called ekāgratā pariṇāma. This happens in the Yogi's mind. It is the first stage of transformation.

Patañjali started from the highest pariṇāma, then the next level down, and now, in YS III.12, the lowest pariṇāma, ekāgratā. He uses the word śāntoditau to again indicate the same thing: one tendency goes down, becomes weak; another stronger. Śānta means subsiding; uditau means arising. Patañjali uses tulya pratyayau which is similar to cittānvayo in III.9. Pratyaya means citta vritti; tulya means non-changing.

Activities of Antaraṅga Sādhana Lead to Pariṇāmas

YS III.12 refers to dhāranā leading to dhyāna. In dhāranā we try and hold the mind on one object. When the mind wanders we bring it back to the object. It takes effort. When we succeed in staying with the object it is dhyāna. When it becomes a habit, when it becomes effortless it is ekāgratā pariṇāma.

Similarly, we may be able to get into samādhi on an object but, it is only when this becomes an effortless habit, when we have built a new saṃskāra that we have transformed the mind. That is samādhi pariṇāma. The same goes for nirodha pariṇāma, the highest transformation.

It is the activities of antaraṅga sādhana which lead to these changes. It is the practice of antaraṅga sādhana which change the saṁskāras of the mind and completely transform it. This is what leads to pariṇāma.

Three Stages of Transformation – A Progression

From ekāgratā pariṇāma you go to samādhi pariṇāma. From samādhi pariṇāma you go ultimately to nirodha pariṇāma.

First get the capability of ekāgra, then develop the state of samādhi, understand everything about prakriti by using the saṃyama capability. (The understanding of all of prakriti using saṃyama also gives you the siddhis.) Having understood, try to go beyond and ultimately try to see the nature of your own Self. Once that is done, try to stay on course, accumulate the new saṃskāras of ekāgratā, samādhi, and nirodha. Over time the mind becomes completely transformed.

Begin with the first level of transformation. From the first level of transformation you go to the second level of transformation. And, from the second level go to the third level of transformation.

Patañjali divides the process into three stages to indicate that one has to go through all three stages of mental transformation.

Bibliography

[YTSL] Yoga for the Three Stages of Life by Srivatsa Ramaswami

[YBS] Yoga Beneath the Surface by Srivatsa Ramaswami and David Hurwitz

[HA] Yoga Philosophy of Patañjali with Bhāsvatī by Swāmī Hariharānanda Āraṇya

[PH] Patañjali's Yoga Sutras: Based on the Teaching of Srivatsa Ramaswami, by Pamela Hoxsey

[SK] Saṁkhya Kārikā of Īśvara Kṛṣṇa

[HYP] The HaṭhaYogaPradīpikā of Svātmārāma (The Adyar Library)

[BG] The Bhagavadgita

[DD] Sāṁkhya A Prologue to Yoga by Deepti Dutta (Khama Publishers)

44777331R00094

Made in the USA
San Bernardino, CA
23 January 2017